Innovations *in* Occupational Therapy Education

2000

Patricia A. Crist, PhD, OTR/L, FAOTA
Editor

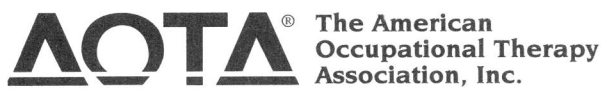

The American Occupational Therapy Association, Inc.
4720 Montgomery Lane
PO Box 31220
Bethesda, Maryland 20824-1220

©2000 by The American Occupational Therapy Association, Inc. All rights reserved. No part of this book may be reproduced in whole or in part by any means without permission.

Disclaimers
This publication is designed to provide accurate and authoritative information in regard to the subject matter covered. It is sold or distributed with the understanding that the publisher is not engaged in rendering legal, accounting, or other professional service. If legal advice or other expert assistance is required, the services of a competent professional person should be sought.
—*From the Declaration of Principles jointly adopted by the American Bar Association and a Committee of Publishers and Associations*

It is the objective of The American Occupational Therapy Association to be a forum for free expression and interchange of ideas. The opinions expressed by the contributors to this work are their own and not necessarily those of either the editors or The American Occupational Therapy Association.

ISBN 1-56900-163-4
Printed in the United States of America.

Table of Contents

IOTE Editorial Board *v*

Foreword

Theory to Practice in Occupational Therapy Education *vii*
 Charlotte Brasic Royeen

Preface *ix*
 Patricia A. Crist

Aim and Scope *xi*

Fieldwork

Brief: A Community Service Learning Approach to Level I Fieldwork: An Investment in the Future *1*
 Marjorie E. Scaffa, Nancy Van Slyke, Donna M. Wooster

Brief: Success of Level II Fieldwork: The Student's Perspective *7*
 Kathleen A. Hughes, Shelia M. Mangold, Stephanie L. Thuss, Steven M. Buckley, and Joanna K. Lennon

Instructional Methods

Modifying the Traditional Classroom in Response to Students' Learning Styles and Sensorimotor Needs *20*
 Susan Bazyk, Glenn Goodman

Understanding the Nature of Process *33*
 Terra Ruppert

Developing a Language for Discussing Writing: Composition in Occupational Therapy? *46*
 Jane Detweiler, Claudia Peyton

Special Section on Problem-Based Learning and Clinical Reasoning

A Review of the Problem-Based Learning Literature in Occupational Therapy *61*
 Lori Caterina, Perri Stern

Essentials for Successful Integration of Problem-Based Learning in Occupational Therapy Curricula *78*
 Betsy VanLeit, Terry K. Crowe, Robert Waterman

Outside of the Textbook: Improving Reasoning and Changing Attitudes About Mental Disabilities   *95*
> Elizabeth Cara

Brief: Pilot Investigation: Evaluation of Clinical Reflection and Reasoning Before and After Workshop Intervention   *107*
> Charlotte Brasic Royeen, Keli Mu, Kate Barrett, Aimee J. Luebben

Academic Leadership

Calls for Reform: A Conceptual Review of Educational Purpose in Occupational Therapy   *116*
> Barb Hooper

Introducing an Awareness of Cultural Diversity Into an Established Curriculum   *134*
> Diana M. Bailey

Brief: Processes for Admission to Occupational Therapy Programs: A Performance-Based Model   *146*
> Lillian Kaplan

Expanding the Utility of Scholarly Activity: Invited Articles   *156*

Establishing Links With Continued Education   *159*
> Suzanne M. Peloquin

Establishing Links With Clinical and Management Functions   *166*
> Beatriz C. Abreu

Establishing Links With Graduate Education   *173*
> Janette K. Schkade

Information for Authors   *178*

IOTE Editorial Board

1998–2000
Alfred G. Bracciano, EdD, OTR
Caroline Robinson Brayley, PhD, OTR/L, FAOTA
Vera-Jean Clark-Brown, MS, L/OTR
Cynthia L. Creighton, PhD, OTR/L
Nancy Lee Hollins, MS, OTR
Aimee J. Luebben, EdD, OTR/L, FAOTA
Anne Cronin Mosey, PhD, OTR, FAOTA
Annette M. Port, COTA
Wendy Starnes, OTR/L
Perri Stern, EdD, OTR

1998–2001
Ellen S. Cohn, ScD, OTR/L, FAOTA
Teru A. Creel, MS, OTR/L
Nedra P. Gillette, ScD(Hon), MEd, OTR, FAOTA
Caryn R. Johnson, MS, OTR/L, FAOTA
Scott D. McPhee, DrPH, MS, MPA, OTR, FAOTA
Susan Cook Merrill, MA, OTR/L
Shirley Peganoff O'Brien, MS, OTR/L, FAOTA
Peggy Owens, MA, OTR/L, FAOTA
Barbara A. Schell, PhD, OT, FAOTA
Janette K. Schkade, PhD, OTR, FAOTA
Mary P. Taugher, PhD, FAOTA
Louise R. Thibodaux, MA, OTR/L, FAOTA
Kay F. Walker, PhD, FAOTA

1999–2002
Marcia Gevelinger Bastian, MS, OTR
Judith E. Bowen, MPA, OTR
Marcia Clinton, COTA/L
Toby Ballou Hamilton, MPH, OTR/L
Debra Lindstrom-Hazel, PhD(c), OTR
Kristie Koenig, MS, OTR/L
Jennie Q. Lou, MD, MSc, OTR/L
Cathy Nielson, MPH, OT/L, FAOTA
Marian Struck, MA, OTR/L
George S. Tomlin, PhD, OT/L
Donna Whitehouse, MHA, OTR

Theory to Practice in Occupational Therapy Education

Charlotte Brasic Royeen

Education and practice in occupational therapy is an art. It is not exact, nor is it inflexible. What makes therapy more than just an art, however, is the science that each of us as practitioners brings to education and to practice. But how do we carry science with us? How can we hold so many facts in our minds? We cannot. In my experience, the master clinician brings his or her "science" to bear in a clinical situation through the use of theory. In other words, theory or a "scheme or system of ideas" (Bothamley, 1993, p. vii) serves as the scientific guide for a practitioner to implement the art of therapy. Similarly, I believe that master teachers use theory or system of ideas as a scientific guide to facilitate the art of teaching and student learning.

According to Bothamley (1993), theory is not only that which is clear in basic science, but also it is that which is somewhat "hazy" (p. vii) in the arts. Theory is the area that allows for guidance by principles and methods. Indeed, that is how I have seen master clinicians and master teachers use theory. Theoretical principles guide their words, thoughts, and actions.

Theory is a "frame of reference that helps humans to understand their world and to function in it" (Chen, 1990, p. 17). I argue that theory is additionally the frame of reference that allows practitioners to understand a given therapeutic encounter and to make sense of it. Similarly, theory may help an educator to understand better a student's given learning experience, to make sense of it, and to better plan for future learning activities.

Sometimes theories are not fully developed, either in the sense defined by basic science or in the more flexible sense defined by the arts. In such cases, conceptual models or conceptual frameworks are often the precursor to a more fully developed theory. In either case, however, a conceptual model or a theory can and should guide practice. It should likewise guide education in occupational therapy.

The articles in this annual relate to conceptual models, frameworks, and theories in many ways.

- Scaffa, Van Slyke, and Wooster apply a community service learning model to fieldwork education.
- Hughes, Mangold, Thuss, Buckley, and Lennon bring participants' views to

educational perspectives in the success of Level II fieldwork.
- Bazyk and Goodman apply sensorimotor theory and learning style to instructional design in the educational environment.
- Ruppert discusses a process and a mechanism of educational activity.
- Detweiler and Peyton present a conceptual model for how to talk about composition in occupational therapy.
- Caterina and Stern synthesize a review of a theoretical approach to learning: problem-based learning.
- VanLeit, Crowe, and Waterman discuss what makes the theoretical model of problem-based learning work.
- Cara addresses how to change attitudes about mental health disabilities.
- Royeen, Mu, Barrett, and Luebben present research on quantitative evaluation of clinical reasoning and reflection.
- Hooper presents a conceptual model of educational purpose in occupational therapy.
- Bailey summarizes a model for how to introduce cultural diversity into existing curricula.
- Kaplan gives us a performance-based model for occupational therapy admissions.
- Peloquin, Abreu, and Schkade each provide a unique view about scholarship within occupational therapy.

This collection of theoretical and empirical work on theory and conceptual models is a superb foundation for continuing educational research in occupational therapy.

The goal of this annual is to provide a forum for scholarly research and reflection on education in occupational therapy. Through this forum, we can disseminate existing educational theory and research in occupational therapy and report new educational innovations in occupational therapy education. Such a groundwork fosters implementation, evaluation, and development of theory in occupational therapy education.

The goal of the AOTA Education Special Interest Section (EDSIS) is to promote networking among educators in occupational therapy. I hope that this text promotes discussion and interaction among you and your colleagues. If so, we will meet, in part, the important mission of the EDSIS.

References

Bothamley, J. (1993). *Dictionary of theories.* London: Gale Research International.

Chen, H. (1990). *Theory-driven evaluations.* Newbury Park, CA: Sage.

Fawcett, J. (1992). *The relationship of theory and research* (3rd ed.). Philadelphia: F. A. Davis.

Charlotte Brasic Royeen, PhD, OTR, is Associate Dean for Research and Professor, Department of Occupational Therapy, School of Pharmacy and Allied Health Professions, Creighton University, Omaha, Nebraska.

Preface

Patricia A. Crist

Welcome to *Innovations in Occupational Therapy Education 2000* (IOTE). This is the second year that the American Occupational Therapy Association (AOTA) has published this annual review for occupational therapy education. The mission of this annual is to provide a collection of innovative educational practices for academic and fieldwork educators in our field. Readers of IOTE are persons in our profession who strive for educational excellence in their roles. We value education and are enchanted by learning and the merit of quality teaching in the classroom, laboratory, clinic, and community. We carefully structure learning to achieve outcomes and bask when unexpected "teachable moments" arise. We strive to use "best practices." IOTE authors willingly share their experiences to reach our common goal. Of course, we strive to be educators in service to the growth of our profession.

We value what our customers (students) say about their learning experiences. Briefly, I must digress and share a story I recently heard about a professor who received his teaching evaluations and read from one student: "If I have but one more hour to live, I would elect to spend it in your class." He took the evaluation home to show to his wife in recognition of his effort. She, being more skeptical, read closely and noted the asterisk at the end with the word "back" written nearby. On the back, the student had written, "because sitting in your class for one hour feels like eternity!" (Blanck, 1999). The reality is that no matter how hard we work or what we may have done, good educators always strive to improve. IOTE supports this internal value among new and experienced educators. Shared experience and humor are antidotes that keep our educators' spirits thriving.

This has been a year of great success. IOTE is now officially referenced in the *Cumulative Index of Nursing and Allied Health Literature* (CINAHL) because it met CINAHL's peer-review standards. Manuscript submissions nearly doubled from the first to the second year. The applications for editorial review board appointments rose nearly 50%. These indicators support the viability of this publication.

The articles contained in this edition provide both innovative ideas that have been implemented and studies documenting the effectiveness of highly lauded or emerging educational practices in the classroom and in fieldwork. As an educator, I am increasingly aware of the limited studies in occupational therapy education that have their basis in educational theory or that test educational approaches ultimately to provide science to couple with our art. Thus, this annual review hopes to change the current state of practice. Innovative, artful approaches warrant documentation. At some point, this art should lead to researchable questions answered through scientific study to substantiate promise and application. Thus, we will have come "full circle" between the art and science of educational practices. Problem-based learning approaches are following this path. I concur with the argument that not all artful practice is testable through scientific approaches. Regardless, if academic education and fieldwork education are to advance, then we must subject our approaches to rigor. Thus, in this edition, creators of innovative approaches provide some form of outcome statements to substantiate their goal or results. More established approaches go beyond description to provide comparative or supportive data. Thus, IOTE can bring new ideas forward while creating a body of knowledge regarding the best practices in occupational therapy education.

I was pleased that we received the first articles regarding occupational therapy assistant education and that IOTE is able to publish one of these. Instructional method articles remained strong, and we noted an increase in administrative leadership articles. As Editor, I sought the publication of the adapted text from a workshop on clinical scholarship presented in Indianapolis. The information warranted wider dissemination because their approach showed not only how to add scholarship to daily full-time work but also how to blend it creatively with current work activities. Many educators are now looking for ways to implement the new *Educational Standards* (Accreditation Council for Occupational Therapy Education, 1999) of practice for occupational therapy education and are pondering the effect of the entry-level master's degree on fieldwork.

I thank the editorial board members who served this year. I extend a special note of gratitude to the founding editorial board members whose duties are completed with the publication of this second edition. These members accepted 2-year appointments initially to implement the rotation plan. As members of the founding board (along with the 1998–2001 members), they were instrumental in establishing and implementing the review process and in bringing the first two volumes to press. The editorial board is the heart of the peer-review process.

References

American Council for Occupational Therapy Education. (1999). *Educational standards*. Bethesda, MD: Author.

Blanck, P. D. (1999). *The unintended consequences of the Americans With Disabilities Act*. Presentation and discussion at the 13th Annual National Disability Management Conference and Exhibit, October 29, 1999, Washington, DC.

Patricia A. Crist, PhD, OTR/L, FAOTA is the Founding Editor, IOTE, and Chair and Professor, Department of Occupational Therapy, Duquesne University, Pittsburgh, Pennsylvania.

Aim & Scope

By focusing on practical application and research in occupational therapy education, *Innovations in Occupational Therapy Education* (IOTE) will facilitate the sharing of contemporary educational approaches among academic and fieldwork educators. By highlighting the best practices in education, the annual, peer-reviewed publication will serve as a resource for educators. Over time, this will become a historical document of the developments in occupational therapy education. Content will include but not be limited to

- instructional methods;
- fieldwork process, supervision, and models;
- professional development of educators and students;
- administration of academic and fieldwork programs; and
- comparative or applied research in education.

Manuscripts on these topics, broadly construed, are encouraged.

The sponsorship of IOTE by the American Occupational Therapy Association is an affirmation of its commitment to advancing the practice of education through scholarship and the communication of viable strategies and resources.

This annual review seeks to publish original manuscripts pertaining to academic and fieldwork education. Manuscripts on a broad range of subjects of potential interest to occupational therapy educators will be considered. Of particular interest are manuscripts that

- demonstrate the value and effectiveness of instructional models and methodologies during fieldwork and academic activities;
- describe contemporary learning approaches by using innovative technology, methods, or resources to promote critical thinking, clinical reasoning, and skill acquisition;
- advance the conceptual basis for the practice of occupational therapy education;
- propose inventive approaches to instructing students in roles including, but not limited to, scholarship, consultation, case management, management, and leadership, as well as professional socialization to the practitioner role in general;
- provide a forum to discuss approaches to educational management and leadership; and
- support the development of faculty members, fieldwork educators, scholars, and academic leaders.

Additionally, scholarly dialogue is encouraged through Letters to the Editor and invited Commentary. Occasionally, the editor will select discussants to critique accepted manuscripts, and such commentary will be published after the designated articles. Readers are welcome to submit thoughtful letters to the editor pertaining to content published in IOTE. Other features include Briefs, which presents concise summaries of new educational approaches; Reviews, which features amplified summaries of educational approaches; and Commentaries, which presents scholarly argument of an education-related view or emerging issue.

Full-length manuscripts are evaluated through a blind review process, and selection is made on the basis of relevance to the profession, scientific merit, timeliness, and scholarly excellence. All contributors are required to assign exclusive copyright to The American Occupational Therapy Association, and assurance must be given that manuscripts are not under consideration for publication elsewhere. Potential contributors should consult submission guidelines published in this volume under "Information for Authors."

FIELDWORK

Brief
A Community Service Learning Approach to Level I Fieldwork: An Investment in the Future

Marjorie E. Scaffa
Nancy Van Slyke
Donna M. Wooster

Marjorie E. Scaffa, PhD, OTR, FAOTA, is Chairperson, Nancy Van Slyke, EdD, OTR, is Academic Fieldwork Coordinator, and Donna M. Wooster, MS, OTR, BCP, is Assistant Professor, Department of Occupational Therapy, University of South Alabama, Mobile, Alabama.

Community service learning, an educational method of active participation through service, has gained national recognition through federal funding programs and foundation grants and is part of various college curricula. The community service learning approach is consistent with occupational therapy's philosophical base and guiding principles. It provides a unique opportunity to meet and expand the profession's objectives and to inform the public about occupational therapy services. This article explores the basic tenets of community service learning and why it is an appropriate educational strategy in occupational therapy; describes a model of Level I fieldwork that uses this approach; and discusses the benefits to students, the occupational therapy program, and the community.

Health care in the United States is going through dramatic upheaval, with changes in health care delivery and health care financing. These changes directly and indirectly affect the profession of occupational therapy in numerous ways. One of the ways that managed care will affect occupational therapy relates to the settings in which services will be provided. A greater number of occupational therapy practitioners will be providing services in the community because of the downsizing of hospitals and decreased lengths of stay for patients. A report by the Agency for Health Care Policy and Research (1996) indicated that the shifting use of health care services across demographic groups and the trend toward community-based systems of care will have important implications for the delivery of occupational therapy services in the near future.

Community-based practice requires a different paradigm, a somewhat different set of skills, and a different perspective of one's role than those that traditional practice in inpatient settings requires. Through community service learning, students have an opportunity to observe real persons with occupational dysfunctions in community settings and to develop new concepts about and approaches to the delivery of occupational therapy services.

Community Service Learning

Community service learning is an educational method by which students learn through participation in planned community service activities that

- meet actual community needs and are integrated into the academic curriculum (they are not merely added to a course);
- provide opportunities for students to apply the skills learned in the classroom to real-life situations;
- provide opportunities for reflection, leadership development, and discussion; and

- foster a sense of care, concern, and compassion for the human community.

The effects of community service learning listed below appear to be broad based and enduring (Conrad & Hedin, 1982, 1991; Giles & Eyler, 1994; Markus, Howard, & King, 1993; Sankaran, Cinelli, McConatha, & Carson, 1995; Wilson, 1974). Service-based learning appears to

- foster open-mindedness;
- increase awareness of one's own values, beliefs, and attitudes;
- increase problem-solving ability;
- increase empathy;
- be as effective as traditional instruction in conveying knowledge;
- increase self-efficacy and enhance the belief that one can make a difference in other persons' lives;
- increase one's sense of social and personal responsibility (which is an important aspect of ethical behavior);
- enhance communication skills;
- reinforce the development of professional behaviors;
- inculcate a healthy work ethic; and
- enable students to evaluate their strengths and weaknesses.

In addition, several potential benefits of community service learning are specific to the discipline of occupational therapy. Community service learning can increase students' understanding of the role of occupational therapy in community-based settings, provide an opportunity to integrate theory with practice, and create networking opportunities with professionals in various nonmedical disciplines. Community service learning allows community-based organizations without occupational therapy services to experience occupational therapy firsthand and increases the potential for the development of new job opportunities for occupational therapy practitioners in community-based programs. A service learning experience may influence a student's choice regarding a community-based setting for future practice. Evidence suggests that practitioners trained in institutions choose to work in similar institutions (Weissert, Knott, & Steiber, 1993). Thus, providing students with experiences in community-based practice early in their academic careers is one of the many reasons for using a community service learning approach for Level I fieldwork.

A Community Service Learning Approach for Level I Fieldwork

As the number of traditional clinical sites for fieldwork opportunities becomes more limited, colleges and universities must seek other sites for fieldwork. Affiliation with local volunteer agencies can enable occupational therapy programs to provide high-quality, supervised, experiential learning opportunities that enhance academic course objectives while reinforcing volunteerism, which is an important aspect of professional development.

Community sites that have an expressed interest in fieldwork education and programs that enhance the learning experience are optimal. Various community facilities can provide community service learning experiences relevant to occupational therapy students, including

- child development programs,
- YMCA and YWCA facilities,
- senior citizens centers,
- senior wellness programs,
- assisted living centers,
- preschools for children with sensory impairments,
- alcohol and drug treatment programs,
- independent living centers,
- sheltered workshops,
- home health care agencies,
- hospice programs,
- local businesses, and
- homeless shelters.

Acquiring a list of United Way agencies in the local community can be an excellent first step in identifying potential sites for community service learning.

At the University of South Alabama in Mobile, community service learning activities have varied among fieldwork experiences; however, each experience has included tasks to complete at the community-based site. Typical learning activities have included weekly entries in reflective journals, observation summaries, checklists, client interviews, evaluations, intervention plans, and development and implementation of group activities.

Students must identify and address a need of the community organization to which they are assigned during each service learning experience. For the first fieldwork placement, the course instructor meets with community agencies, identifies needs, and creates a list of potential projects from which students can choose. For subsequent fieldwork placements, students conduct a needs evaluation and determine appropriate projects to meet the identified needs of individual clients, staff members, or the setting. A few examples of projects completed include

- constructing switch toys for children with disabilities;
- developing and implementing a health promotion program for persons being treated for substance abuse problems;

- creating and adapting opportunities for participation in horticulture;
- assisting persons with terminal illnesses to create life story books or videos;
- making environmental modifications for persons with visual impairments or physical disabilities;
- building adaptive equipment;
- creating training programs for agency and organization staff members; and
- designing, implementing, and training clients of mental health services to operate a small store.

Considerations in Developing Community Service Learning Strategies

Although access to various age groups and programs has greatly enhanced learning opportunities, volunteering in community organizations has not been without limitations. Professionals of varying backgrounds (e.g., social work, medicine [psychiatry], nursing, physical and speech therapy, counseling) provide supervision at most of these sites. In addition, because many of these programs are not for profit and are often funded through the United Way, resources for supplies and equipment are limited. The most common complaints of students include lack of occupational therapy role models (because the supervisors are often not occupational therapy practitioners), lack of structured intervention programs, and poor availability of appropriate supplies and equipment. Faculty member concerns about using service learning in community-based sites include

- the amount of time required to orient supervisors to fieldwork objectives, expectations, and administration of student performance evaluations;
- the additional classroom time necessary to help students process observations; and
- the potential roles and functions of occupational therapy within the various community sites.

All involved parties have benefited in many ways from using a community service learning approach to Level I fieldwork in the curriculum. The occupational therapy department gains positive visibility within the university and community. The agencies and programs that collaborate with the program in providing this experience for students receive high-quality volunteers with some fairly sophisticated skills, and the students gain knowledge of and experience in community-based practice settings. The success of this fieldwork model depends on numerous factors, including the students' attitudes and motivation; good communication among the academic fieldwork coordinator, individual faculty members, and the supervisors on site; and the clarity of the fieldwork objectives and assignments.

Summary

Major changes in health care have necessitated changes in the way that educational programs train occupational therapy students. A different paradigm for both academic and fieldwork education is necessary. Educational programs can no longer rely on hospital-based sites for clinical education. Students must learn to function in community-based sites. Level I fieldwork experiences that involve the principles of community service learning can be a major investment in the future of the occupational therapy profession.

References

Agency for Health Care Policy and Research. (1996). *Health care and market reform: Workforce implications for occupational therapy* (Report prepared by the American Occupational Therapy Association). Washington, DC: U.S. Government Printing Office.

Conrad, D., & Hedin, D. (1982). The impact of experiential education on adolescent development. *Child and Youth Services, 4,* 57–76.

Conrad, D., & Hedin, D. (1991). School-based community service: What we know from research and theory. *Phi Delta Kappan, 72,* 743–749.

Giles, D. E., & Eyler, J. (1994). The impact of a college community service laboratory on students' personal, social and cognitive outcomes. *Journal of Adolescence, 17,* 327–339.

Markus, G. B., Howard, J. P., & King, D. C. (1993). Integrating community service and classroom instruction enhances learning: Results from an experiment. *Educational Evaluation and Policy Analysis, 15,* 410–419.

Sankaran, G., Cinelli, B., McConatha, D., & Carson, L. (1995). Voluntarism: An investment in preparing health professionals for the future. *Journal of Health Education, 26*(1), 58–60.

Weissert, C., Knott, J., & Steiber, B. (1993). *Health professions education reform: Understanding and explaining states' policy options.* East Lansing, MI: Michigan State University, Department of Political Science and the Institute for Public Policy and Social Research.

Wilson, T. C. (1974). *An alternative community-based school education program and student political development.* Unpublished doctoral dissertation, University of Southern California, Los Angeles.

FIELDWORK

Brief Success of Level II Fieldwork: The Student's Perspective

Kathleen A. Hughes
Sheila M. Mangold
Stephanie L. Thuss
Steven M. Buckley
Joanna K. Lennon

Kathleen A. Hughes, OTR/L, is Occupational Therapist, Inpatient Rehabilitation, Sheila M. Mangold, OTR/L, is Occupational Therapist, Inpatient Rehabilitation, Stephanie L. Thuss, OTR/L, is Occupational Therapist, School-Based Practice, Steven M. Buckley, OTR/L, is Occupational Therapist, School-Based Practice, and Joanna K. Lennon, OTR/L, is Occupational Therapist, Occupational Therapy Department, College Misericordia, Dallas, Pennsylvania.

The purpose of this study was to discover the characteristics necessary for a student to be successful in Level II fieldwork. The study used a phenomenological design. The informants were persons who had successfully completed Level II fieldwork, as determined by their Level II fieldwork educator, in accordance with the American Occupational Therapy Association's Fieldwork Evaluation for the Occupational Therapist. *The data were gathered from interviews with the informants. Their responses were analyzed by using both content and thematic analysis. The results indicate the importance of the following characteristics: interpersonal interactions, the role of the supervisor, a structured environment, other students, personality, educational background, and time management. The results may have implications for occupational therapy students' fieldwork and practice. Furthermore, this study highlights the importance of the fieldwork educator as a role model and mentor.*

Success of Level II Fieldwork: The Student's Perspective

Occupational therapy fieldwork is a major component in the preparation of the occupational therapy practitioner. The purpose of fieldwork is to provide the student with opportunities to apply and refine knowledge from the academic setting in the practice setting (American Occupational Therapy Association [AOTA], 1996). The purpose of this research was to discover student perspectives of the characteristics relevant to successful completion of Level II fieldwork. The research question guiding this investigation was: What factors enable students to be successful during Level II fieldwork? In accordance with the AOTA's (1987) *Fieldwork Evaluation for the Occupational Therapist*, the researchers have defined *success* as completely satisfying the requirements concerning the Level II fieldwork experience. In addition, the researchers defined *outstanding manner* as performance exceeding the fieldwork educator's expectations of the student's performance, judgment, and attitude regarding the fieldwork experience (AOTA, 1987).

Rationale for Using Qualitative Research

Few studies have investigated the topic of success in Level II fieldwork by using the qualitative method, specifically the phenomenological design (Mickan, 1995; Tompson & Ryan, 1996). Related studies have used quantitative methods (Best, 1994; Donohue, 1995). The researchers believed that the inductive approach was appropriate because prior research may not have considered an emic perspective (i.e., one that uses the words of the informants to gain insight into the phenomenon of student success).

Researchers' Position in the Study

The five researchers were entry-level occupational therapy master's degree students at the time of the study. Successful completion of Level II fieldwork was an area of interest because of the researchers' anticipation of this component of their educational program.

Importance to Occupational Therapy

Identifying what enables students to succeed during fieldwork can enhance student preparation for this component of the educational experience. In addition, the information that informants provided identified aspects of the Level II fieldwork experience that fieldwork educators can use to strengthen their position as role models or mentors.

Literature Review

An accepted belief is that "occupational therapy, in the tradition of the medical model of education, relies on clinical fieldwork to provide students with experiences necessary for professional practice" (Meyers, 1989, p. 348). Level II fieldwork is a common, recurring subject of interest in the occupational therapy literature (Best, 1994; Donohue, 1995; Mickan, 1995; Tompson & Ryan, 1996). Fieldwork is the gateway for students to gain experience within the clinical setting, thereby increasing the opportunities for them to be successful practitioners.

Best (1994) examined the relationship of fieldwork success and student grade point average and found that grades are not a strong predictor of student fieldwork performance. This study suggests that further research should focus on variables not specifically related to grades. Best (1994) cites many authors who have suggested the need for further exploration of this subject.

In another quantitative study, Donohue (1995) focused on the development of specific traits that entry-level occupational therapy students acquire from the first year of their educational careers to the completion of their Level II fieldwork experiences. Donohue stated that occupational therapy curricula may have an effect on the performance of students during fieldwork. Gough's California Psychological Inventory (CPI) (as cited in Donohue, 1995) measured personality traits of students before and after their participation in academic and clinical experiences. The purpose of the CPI was to determine the change in personality traits and how academic or fieldwork experiences affected the personality changes. According to Donohue, the students' scores in 13 of 18 personality trait areas, such as responsibility, well-being, and intellectual efficiency, improved after fieldwork, which indicates that "professional socialization may be fostered by participation in an occupational therapy academic and clinical curriculum" (p. 708).

By using a qualitative approach, Mickan (1995) investigated the importance of theoretical knowledge and student preparation for pediatric fieldwork. The two areas that were vital to student performance were student knowledge of course material and professional and personal interaction skills. The main findings of this study were that each fieldwork experience is individual and that each student must be responsible for his or her own learning.

The qualitative research of Tompson and Ryan (1996) focused on the professional socialization that students acquire during their fieldwork experiences. Their study concentrated on the student's ability to gain a clear understanding of practice through the fieldwork experience. Tompson and Ryan stated that, although this study focused on students and their professional socialization, further exploration is necessary to obtain more information regarding students and their perceptions about fieldwork.

Prior research did not specifically investigate the perspective of students regarding their performance during fieldwork. Therefore, we considered this topic to be an appropriate avenue of research for this project.

Method

Introduction to Type of Design and Rationale for Choice

The researchers chose a phenomenological design. By using this approach, the researchers' goals were to gain information from the informants on what they believe made them successful during their Level II fieldwork experiences.

Number and Role of the Researchers

Each of the five researchers conducted an in-person interview with at least one informant. The individual researchers independently performed content analysis of his or her interview(s). The researchers and the research chairperson (Grace Sheldon-Fisher, EdD, OTR/L) performed thematic analysis collectively.

Informants

Informants were persons who had successfully completed a Level II fieldwork experience in an outstanding manner within the past 2 years.

The researchers obtained a list of fieldwork coordinators representing the northeastern region of the United States through an independent party. Each randomly selected fieldwork coordinator received a packet of information describing the study and requesting that he or she forward the packet to a fieldwork educator. We then requested that each educator nominate a fieldwork student who had satisfied the criteria for the study. The educator forwarded the information to the student. The nominated student contacted the researchers via a toll-free telephone number if he or she was interested in participating in the study.

Considering the nature of the research, the most appropriate way to acquire information regarding the success of Level II fieldwork experiences was to obtain information directly from the informants. By using nominated informants, the researchers had assurance that the informants had met the criteria for success.

Data Collection

The researchers conducted individualized personal interviews. The informants responded to one open-ended question that allowed them to express their perceptions about the fieldwork experience on an individual level. The open-ended question was: Describe what has made you successful in your Level II fieldwork experience. The researchers used probes as necessary to clarify and expand on the information that the informants offered. Other pertinent information that the informants provided was demographic information, including age, gender, time elapsed since fieldwork experience, type of educational therapy program (bachelor's degree or master of science degree), and specialty area of concentration during the fieldwork experience. Each informant selected a pseudonym to ensure confidentiality.

The information provided during the interview was recorded on audiotape and transcribed verbatim. The interviews ranged in length from 30 min to 60 min. The researchers conducted content analysis of the individual transcripts to identify categories of important data. The researchers and research chairperson then conducted cross-transcript thematic analysis to derive themes.

Results

Informants

Susan is a 22-year-old woman who earned an entry-level master's degree in occupational therapy from a small, suburban, Catholic liberal arts college. The fieldwork experience she discussed was in the area of pediatrics. Eight months had elapsed since the end of her Level II fieldwork experience.

David is a 22-year-old man who completed his fieldwork experience in the mental health setting approximately 5 months before the interview. He is a graduate of a small, suburban, liberal arts college where he earned his bachelor of science degree in occupational therapy.

Abby is a 22-years-old woman from a small, urban university where she earned her bachelor of science degree in occupational therapy. She finished a psychosocial Level II fieldwork experience 5 days before her participation in this study.

Lisa, a 27-years-old woman, received an entry-level master's degree in occupational therapy from an urban university. Fourteen months had elapsed since her fieldwork experience. The concentration of her fieldwork was physical disabilities.

Ann is a 24-year-old woman who has been a practicing pediatric occupational therapist for approximately 2 years. She is a graduate of a small, suburban, liberal arts college where she earned her bachelor of science degree in occupational therapy.

The Emerging Themes

Analysis of informant interviews yielded seven themes that informants deemed vital to successful completion of Level II fieldwork assignments.

Interpersonal interactions facilitated student success. An important finding was that of interpersonal interactions. Susan, David, Abby, and Lisa believed that their ability to communicate honestly with their supervisors and patients assisted them in successfully completing their fieldwork experiences.

Susan discussed how honest communication helped her to have a more open relationship with her supervisor. She talked about instances when she was "in over my head" and had many assignments and responsibilities. Susan discussed her feelings with her supervisor, and together they found ways to help her make her experience more manageable.

David said that being "an effective communicator and being an assertive communicator…with both my patients and my supervisor" contributed to his success. He spoke of an experience in which a patient did not seem to be reacting well to him or his intervention approach. When David communicated his frustrations to his supervisor, they developed a plan to improve this situation. David believed that building a good rapport with patients and using patient-directed goals for intervention were essential to his success during fieldwork.

Abby believed that communicating her needs to her supervisor made her successful. She stated, "I guess the more I got into [my fieldwork], I realized that communication was very, very important just to the success of your fieldwork and getting the job done right." Abby believed that being comfortable in communicating her needs to her supervisor was essential, as was her supervisor's comfort in being open and honest with Abby. She mentioned that open communication assisted her in having a more positive attitude, and the feedback received from her supervisor "helped me to do my job better."

Lisa explained how open communication with her supervisor and with the other staff members improved the quality of her learning experience during fieldwork. Lisa stated, "There was always someone there who could answer my questions, no matter how detailed or specific it was."

The fieldwork supervisor acted as a guide and mentor. Another prominent finding was the importance of the supervisor's role in the fieldwork process. Several informants attributed their success to the fact that their fieldwork supervisor played an important role in their professional development.

Lisa and Ann were convinced that their supervisors' knowledge was an important aspect of the fieldwork experience. Lisa stated, "It was her fantastic knowledge base…if she didn't know something, there was always someone in the department who did; she always helped me find out where to go." Ann said, "My supervisor was very helpful…she spent a lot of time teaching me different things that I didn't learn in school or that I may have touched on in school, but she went into more detail about it." Lisa described her supervisor as a guide. She stated, "She gave me a lot of guidance in the beginning when I did not have the experience…until I felt comfortable." In addition, Ann commented, "She also spent a lot of time every week going over things…I felt it was above and beyond what…her role as a supervisor would have been." According to Ann, her supervisor's experience in the field also contributed to her success in fieldwork. Ann mentioned, "She has been working for…8 or 9 years at the time…she had a lot of different experiences…she had worked in several places beforehand."

Susan described her daily meetings with her supervisor as important to her fieldwork experience. She stated that they had "a couple minutes to…process the day, this is what happened today, these are the questions I have." Susan and her supervisor met weekly for 1 hr. Susan explained, "We had 10 questions that we answered…from what diagnoses did you see this week to…how well are you performing in your therapy." Susan believed that the meeting was helpful and stated, "[The meeting] let you reflect on the week and say…I saw this child and I really don't think that I did anything that was too beneficial. Maybe I could try this…or suggestions for trying something new." In addition to the daily and weekly meetings, Susan and her supervisor completed an evaluation that the facility required. She stated, "This helped a lot because there was question by question…filling out what helped and what didn't help…identifying areas where I thought I could use…more supervision and [she] could say areas she thought…I could do a little better."

According to David, his student–supervisor experience was a "two-way street." He commented, "A fieldwork experience…[is] half the student and half the supervisor…if you have a really good supervisor, I think you can have a good fieldwork experience." David explained that his supervisor encouraged him to learn about himself during fieldwork. David stated, "She's really concerned with a lot of self-discovery, more than just [occupational therapy]…how do I feel about working with the mental health population…how do I deal with someone who's been discharged and…has come back."

A structured educational environment for fieldwork helped students become all they could be. The structure of the educational environment was a domain for some students in their Level II fieldwork experiences. Susan, Lisa, David, and Ann commented on how a structured educational environment for fieldwork helped them to be successful.

Susan found that the use of a protocol that the facility gave her helped tremendously. She stated, "I felt more comfortable with how to treat each diagnosis because I actually had a written protocol for each one…[it was] something to follow from the minute you walked in the door to the minute that you...looked at the chart." She spoke of the orientation process that the facility provided and stated, "The first couple weeks I touched upon each area, which...let me get comfortable with what was going on...that was part of the way that they had their program set up, so they didn't throw you into treating patients."

Lisa stated, "My first week here we had a really low census, so I think I must have had about five in-services a day...at the same time they were showing me how to do visual-perceptual tests, sensory tests...they reviewed everything, from different blood pressure and pulse to cardiac precautions." She further stated, "The department gave me a three-ring binder that had different sections in it, and it started out with hospital policies, and my supervisor put together a notebook; it had everything that I needed."

Ann commented on the in-service presentations she attended during her experience and stated, "The whole staff was very helpful because they had...an in-service for the students where the different therapists who had a specialty in different areas would teach us."

David spoke of orientation programs in his interview, stating, "I think they had a lot of student-oriented programs...there was a very good student program...they always want to get new people in."

Other students acted as a support system. Another finding showed the importance of working with other students. Lisa, Susan, Abby, and David all believed in the common bond of working with other students because they were all encountering similar experiences. They were able to express frustrations to the other students that they were unable to express to their supervisors.

Lisa commented, "I thought...with the other students it was really good, just to ask questions that maybe I didn't feel comfortable asking my supervisor." Lisa spoke of how working with occupational therapy and physical therapy students assisted her in learning how the two professions work together. Other informants indicated that the presence of other students was helpful. Susan said that other students provided "a friend."

The informants believed that students were good resources for each other in that they provided additional intervention ideas and helped one another view different therapy techniques and conditions in a new way. Abby said that she was "able to bounce ideas off of somebody else, kind of a neutral party, somebody who wasn't totally in charge but kind of at the same level as I was." David stated, "I think students who are together on a fieldwork are pretty supportive of one another; they're going through the same thing you are, so they're really helpful."

Personality helped students rise to the top. Another finding that the informants identified as helping them to succeed in their Level II fieldwork experiences was personality. The informants spoke of their individual personalities and of their personal learning styles as components that helped them to succeed. David identified having an open mind as being an asset during his fieldwork experience. He stated, "I think the more open you are to try new things, the more you will get out of it…just try to make the best of the situation because, obviously, I can't control everything in a fieldwork situation."

Abby spoke of her attitude as an asset during her fieldwork experience. She stated, "What made me most successful was my attitude. I was positive about going to my fieldworks and wanting to do a good job…when my supervisor gave me feedback, that helped my attitude…and [it] made me want to do my job better."

David likewise believed that his attitude was an attribute to his successful completion of Level II fieldwork. He added, "I tried to get something positive out of each fieldwork experience no matter how negative the experience was.…I expect to have a good experience regardless of what setting I'm in."

Informants identified confidence in themselves as being a contributor to their success during Level II fieldwork. Susan stated, "I had confidence that what I was doing and my educational background had prepared me for what treatment I was giving…I also didn't hesitate to ask for help…that's something that I also think is very important."

Informants spoke about the importance of personal learning style, such as hands-on and self-directed learning, to attain success during fieldwork. Ann specified how she spent additional preparation time at home reading about different topics. David preferred hands-on learning. He stated, "I like to get in there and really do things and then get some feedback afterwards."

Educational background set the stage for student success. Educational background, or schooling, was an influencing factor for attaining success in the Level II fieldwork experience. The informants referred to various aspects of their educational background, including previous Level I and II fieldwork experiences, general occupational therapy theory course work, and courses specific to the specialty areas of pediatrics and physical disabilities.

Abby stated, "My physical disabilities Level I [fieldwork]…opened my eyes to what an [occupational therapist] does in physical disabilities." Ann, referring to previous Level II fieldwork experiences, commented, "I would say that my other fieldworks probably helped…I kind of already knew how things were going to be and what to expect in terms of requirements." Lisa stated, "Once I started treating patients, I would remember what I had learned in school. I could go back and look through my notes and then…understand what they were trying to tell me." Abby commented, "My school focuses a lot on professional behaviors…being professional…empathetic to your patients, have good communication skills, be organized…there was a big focus [on professional behaviors] throughout our whole college education." Ann discussed general theory as well as course work specific to pediatrics, stating, "The preparation that I got from school, all the theories and backgrounds…learning about what [occupational therapy] is…that was just the foundation for all of my skills." She also stated, "I think [my school] does a good job with the amount of schooling that they give us in pediatrics. We have a couple of pediatric classes and labs. We had a whole class in sensory integration…I think that was helpful because we did get a lot of background in [pediatrics]."

Time management provides essential structure for success. Three informants referred to time management as a skill that contributed to the success of their Level II fieldwork experiences. Susan stated, "I was able to manage my time partly due to my [supervisor]…giving me a set schedule in the beginning and then being able to carry that over when I could develop my own schedule, and partly due to the fact that I remained organized throughout my whole [fieldwork experience]."

In addition, Abby stated, "Working my way through high school and college, I was involved in a lot of things that required time management and that definitely carried over to Level II [fieldwork] because you had to worry about treating patients, doing your paperwork, planning treatment sessions, and keeping someone's prescription up for services…it required a lot of time management."

Ann stated, "I think that professionally speaking…I treat others with respect…time management, and judgment and all of those things…I don't think that they were ever a problem for me."

Bringing It All Together: The Summary

Each informant related the theme of interpersonal interactions. The informants believed that the supervisors' ability as well as their own to communicate their needs effectively was essential to their success. They commented that, along with strong interpersonal skills, supervisors who offered them guidance and support and met with them consistently facilitated their success. Informants believed that interacting with other students was beneficial because the students acted as support systems and resources. They reported that student orientation and in-service presentations that facilities offered played a role in their success. Informants mentioned that their educational background (especially the skills they learned during Level I fieldwork experiences and occupational therapy course work) was highly valued and necessary. Positive personality, open-mindedness, and awareness of their personal learning style were fundamental to the informants' success during their fieldwork experiences. In addition, they believed that an ability to manage their time was imperative because of the many responsibilities of a fieldwork student. Thus, they identified numerous critical factors as vital to successful completion of Level II fieldwork.

Discussion

Interpretation of Results

On the basis of the information that we derived from the thematic analysis, we recommend that occupational therapy educational programs include course work focusing on interpersonal interaction skills, such as effective communication, professional behaviors, and empathetic values. Factors beyond students' control also influence success during Level II fieldwork experiences. Several informants cited extrinsic factors, such as the fieldwork supervisor and the structured environment of the facility, as irreplaceable facets of this part of their education. Fieldwork educators must be aware of their unique effect on students' fieldwork experiences. Facilities accepting Level II fieldwork students must be open to providing a structured environment to contribute to student learning. Furthermore, fellow students provide a valuable support system.

Time management was an intrinsic skill that the informants believed was essential to their successful experiences. Adequate time management skills allowed students to structure their interactions with patients and supervisors while accomplishing their assignments and responsibilities. The students needed to build on and refine skills associated with time management continually to ensure effective performance during fieldwork placements.

This study clearly illustrates the importance of student personality. Students possessing a positive attitude, self-confidence, and open-mindedness found these attributes to be imperative when interacting with their supervisors, staff members, peers, and patients. This study supports the need for students to identify and understand their learning styles before entering fieldwork. Students should be able to articulate their learning needs to fieldwork educators to gain a more personalized learning experience.

Relationship to the Existing Body of Literature

Herzberg (1994) used a focus discussion group that examined the perspectives of occupational therapy practitioners within the areas of physical disabilities and mental health. She identified teamwork, active experimentation, flexibility, adaptability, and doing as essential to the student fieldwork process. Herzberg's findings support the results of the current investigation in terms of the importance of student–supervisor interaction and student relationships with peers. Furthermore, the concepts of active experimentation, flexibility, adaptability, and doing relate to this study's finding of student personality as essential to successful completion of Level II fieldwork experiences.

Meyers (1989) examined the concept of ideal fieldwork environments in the areas of mental health, adult physical disabilities, and pediatrics. She found that the concepts of supervision, communication, supervisor expertise, and contextual structure were vitally important, with varying emphasis on these areas in the different clinical environments. Meyers' (1989) findings correlate with the results of the present study in that they support the themes of interpersonal interaction, role of the supervisor, structured environment, and possibly other students.

Best (1994) suggested that the student–supervisor relationship influences students' attitudes. He stated that "the high correlation between attitude and performance implies that the quality of the student–supervisor relationship is critical" (Best, 1994, p. 929). This lends further support for the current study's finding of the importance of interpersonal interaction skills of students and supervisors.

Recommendations for Future Research

The current study of the success of Level II fieldwork students was an attempt to clarify the factors contributing to outstanding fieldwork success according to the informants' perspectives. This subject requires further inquiry because we have not fully exhausted it. Further research may include an ethnomethodological study examining student and supervisor relationships, an ethnographic view of occupational therapy students in fieldwork environments, and a phenomenological design comparing the perceptions of occupational therapy assistants and occupational therapists regarding success in the fieldwork experience.

Issues of Trustworthiness

To enhance consistency, the researchers posed the same question to each informant. We achieved triangulation of data sources by conducting interviews with five persons. This contributed to the transferability of the findings. The process of member checking was conducted among researchers to validate the content analysis, which contributed to the level of credibility of the study. The researchers used peer debriefing in multiple dialogue sessions with the researchers and the research chairperson. All data related to this study were available in a secured area to ensure confirmability.

The limitations of this study may include several factors: age, variance in degree attainment, time elapsed since fieldwork completion, biases of fieldwork educators affecting the perception of student success, specialty area of concentration in the fieldwork experience, and differences in the interview style among the five researchers. Each informant was considered outstanding in his or her performance of Level II fieldwork, which possibly reduces the transferability of the results to students who demonstrate average performance. Only four occupational therapy programs were represented in this study, each being located within the northeastern region of the United States.

Implications for the Field of Occupational Therapy

The results of this preliminary study carry implications for occupational therapy fieldwork students from the perspective of these five informants. The results suggest a three-tiered framework applicable to the Level II fieldwork experience. First, the five informants suggested that an interplay of various components, which we identified as the emerging themes of this study, contributed to their individual success. Second, the informants, when faced with the challenges of fieldwork, called on their strengths of flexibility and self-awareness to guide them through the experience. Finally, educators in clinical and academic settings may provide opportunities for students to enhance both professional and personal growth by facilitating a greater level of self-awareness and skill acquisition. Facilities should provide the opportunity for many students to participate in the fieldwork experience simultaneously. ■

Acknowledgments

We thank the informants who participated in this study and generously offered their time, experience, and knowledge regarding this phenomenon. We thank Grace Sheldon-Fisher, EdD, OTR/L, and Beth P. Velde, PhD, OTR/L, for their guidance and support throughout this research study and Ellen McLaughlin, MS, OTR/L, Jeffrey Johnson, PhD, Dawn Evans, OTR/L, and Susan Barry, BS, for their contributions to this process.

References

American Occupational Therapy Association. (1987). *Fieldwork evaluation for the occupational therapist*. Bethesda, MD: Author.

American Occupational Therapy Association. (1996). Statement: Purpose and value of occupational therapy fieldwork education. *American Journal of Occupational Therapy, 50,* 845.

Best, C. E. (1994). A prediction model of performance in Level II fieldwork in physical disabilities. *American Journal of Occupational Therapy, 48,* 926–931.

Donohue, M. V. (1995). A study of the development of traits of entry-level occupational therapy students. *American Journal of Occupational Therapy, 49,* 703–709.

Herzberg, G. L. (1994). The successful fieldwork student: Supervisor perceptions. *American Journal of Occupational Therapy, 48,* 817–823.

Meyers, S. K. (1989). Program evaluation of occupational therapy Level II fieldwork environments: A naturalistic inquiry. *Occupational Therapy Journal of Research, 9,* 347–361.

Mickan, S. M. (1995). Student preparation for pediatric fieldwork. *British Journal of Occupational Therapy, 58,* 239–244.

Tompson, M. M., & Ryan, A. G. (1996). The influence of fieldwork on the professional socialization of occupational therapy students. *British Journal of Occupational Therapy, 9,* 70.

INSTRUCTIONAL METHODS

Modifying the Traditional Classroom in Response to Students' Learning Styles and Sensorimotor Needs

Susan Bazyk
Glenn Goodman

Susan Bazyk, MHS, OTR/L, is Associate Professor, and Glenn Goodman, MOT, OTR/L, is Associate Professor, Occupational Therapy Program, Department of Health Sciences, Cleveland State University, Cleveland, Ohio.

A traditional college classroom was modified with sensorimotor materials to respond to students' individual learning styles and sensorimotor preferences (tactile, oral, proprioceptive, vestibular) to enhance optimal arousal for learning. Classroom modifications were used with second-year occupational therapy students during 8 weeks of class. At the end of the course, students completed a survey documenting their use of the materials. In addition, a pilot study with a quasi-experimental design compared students' self-ratings of arousal in the modified versus traditional classroom at six intervals during a 2-hr class period. Although the results indicate no significant difference between groups in levels of arousal, between-interval comparisons and slope lines suggest a positive cumulative effect from the use of the sensorimotor materials. In addition, the survey results indicate that most students (87.5%) used the sensorimotor items in the modified classroom, with students most often using objects to put into one's mouth, followed by objects to touch and items offering opportunities to move.

The traditional college classroom is generally uniform in design, with solid plastic or wooden desks for students. Almost all classroom furniture is seemingly designed in ways to deny comfort and to promote the need for frequent movement (Dunn & Dunn, 1991). General expectations are that students remain seated at their desks until a break or until the end of class. In addition, professors may or may not allow beverage or food consumption in the classroom. This traditional classroom design assumes that all students prefer a formal setting for learning. In reality, students come to us as a heterogeneous group with different learning styles and sensorimotor requirements for attending and learning. Academicians generally do not consider the effects of the traditional classroom on student attitude, attending, and achievement (Dunn, 1991).

According to Dunn and Dunn's work with learning styles, analytics (i.e., step-by-step sequential processors who concentrate initially on details before gaining a full understanding of concepts) and globals (i.e., persons who require holistic comprehension before learning details) learn in ways that are opposite of each other and require different types of learning environments (Dunn, 1990). Analytics prefer formal learning environments (e.g., traditional desks, uncluttered work surfaces, quiet, florescent lighting), whereas globals prefer informal environments (e.g., softer seats, opportunities to move, background music, reduced lighting). Studies have documented higher achievement in elementary and junior high students with global learning styles when they were permitted to sit on bean bag chairs, soft furniture, or cushions (Hodges, 1985; Shea, 1983).

Numerous studies have measured the effects of matching various instructional strategies with specific learning style patterns in college students (Boulmetis & Sabula, 1996; Dunn & Nelson, 1996; Griggs, Griggs, Dunn, & Ingham, 1994; Lenehan, Dunn, Ingham, Signer, & Murray, 1994). A meta-analytical study of 42 experimental studies conducted between 1980 and 1990 with the Dunn & Dunn Learning Styles Model indicated that instruction responsive to a student's multiple learning style elements can produce greatly increased academic achievement (Dunn, Griggs, Olson, & Beasley, 1995). These instructional strategies focus largely on restructuring how one learns on the basis of one's strongest sensory modality (e.g., vision, auditory, tactile, kinesthetic). For example, when students prefer learning through their auditory sense, they should listen to the professor's lecture before reading and taking notes; on the other hand, visual learners should complete their readings before class (Dunn, 1988). The Dunn & Dunn Learning Styles Model provides suggestions for modifying learning on the basis of individual needs related to noise, light, temperature, seating, oral intake, and time of day (Dunn, & Dunn, 1987). These sensory variables are generally discussed from the perspective of a person's preferences without an emphasis on how sensorimotor input can influence a person's neurobehavioral organization for arousal and attending in the classroom.

Occupational therapy practitioners' understanding of the nervous system and sensory processing can contribute to a fuller understanding of how sensory input may affect one's level of arousal while learning. Williams and Shellenberger (1992), for example, developed the Alert Program for Self-Regulation for children with learning difficulties. They have since adapted this program for adults as well. The Alert Program teaches persons about variations in states of arousal by likening this concept to an engine running too high, too low, or just right for a given task and how to use sensorimotor strategies to self-regulate states of arousal for learning. *Arousal* is the state of the nervous system that influences how alert one feels. To attend, concentrate, and function in a classroom, one must be in an optimal state of arousal for learning. *Self-regulation* involves the ability to attain, maintain, and change arousal appropriately for learning. The Alert Program teaches students how to self-regulate their arousal for learning by using various materials and activities in the classroom to provide sensorimotor input. Sensorimotor strategies include having objects to touch (e.g., Koosh balls [Oddzon, Napa, California]), putting objects into one's mouth (e.g., food items), and having opportunities to move (e.g., sitting on a Move-n-Sit cushion [Ledraplastic, Osoppo, Italy]). Students self-select various sensorimotor strategies on the basis of an analysis of their unique sensorimotor preferences (Williams & Shellenberger, 1992). A review of current literature found no studies exploring the benefits of sensorimotor strategies as described in the Alert Program with college students.

This pilot study is unique in its application of Williams and Shellenberger's (1992) Alert Program to modify a traditional college classroom for optimal student attending and learning. The purpose of this study was to provide occupational therapy students with an opportunity to experience firsthand the use of sensorimotor strategies to self-regulate levels of arousal for learning in the classroom, to compare students' self-ratings of arousal in the modified versus traditional classroom, and to identify trends in student use of the modified classroom materials. A quasi-experimental design compared self-ratings of arousal in the modified versus traditional classroom. A written survey obtained descriptive data regarding student use of the sensorimotor materials in the modified classroom during an 8-week period.

Method

Modified Classroom

Materials that would offer various forms of sensorimotor input were purchased and organized in a cabinet in the project's designated classroom. These materials offer global learners opportunities to create a less formal learning environment (e.g., pillows, fleece throws) and offer all students various sensorimotor experiences on the basis of individual sensory needs. Classroom materials offered students opportunities to move (e.g., Move-n-Sit cushions, pillows), touch (e.g., Koosh balls, squishy and spongy balls, Thera-Band tubing [Hygenic Corp., Akron, Ohio], Klix [Chase Toys, Ventura, California], fleece blankets), and put something into their mouths (e.g., gum, crunchy foods, hard candy, chewy candy, sour gummy worms). Classroom policies for use and maintenance of these materials were posted on the sensorimotor cabinet.

Study Design

A quasi-experimental design compared student levels of arousal for learning in the modified versus traditional classroom. After giving informed consent, 33 second-year occupational therapy students were randomly assigned to either the experimental (modified classroom) or control (traditional classroom) groups. Students did not know whether their group was the experimental or control group. On the day of the study, the principal investigator presented a 2-hr class to each group separately from 8:00 a.m. to 10:00 a.m. (control group) and from 10:00 a.m. to 12:00 noon (experimental group). During the class, the students rated their level of arousal at six different time intervals by using a 10-point Likert scale (0 = drowsy/inattentive, 10 = optimal level of arousal or attentive and alert). The experimental and control groups used the same time intervals for rating arousal (first hour: 20 min, 35 min, and 45 min; second hour: 15 min, 30 min, and 45 min). For this pilot study, the first measure of arousal became baseline data for the students in each group. Both groups had a 10-min break between the first and second hours. Students in the modified classroom received a brief introduction before the lecture on selection and use of the materials in the sensorimotor cabinet on the basis of individual learning style and sensorimotor needs.

Use of the Modified Classroom

After the day of the study, materials in the sensorimotor cabinet were then available to all students for each class period throughout the remainder of the semester (8 weeks). As a part of the course content, students learned about the Dunn & Dunn Learning Styles Model (Dunn, 1990) and the Alert Program for Self-Regulation (Williams & Shellenberger, 1996). In addition, each student completed the Productivity Environmental Preference Survey (Dunn, Dunn, & Price, 1989) and the Sensory-Motor Preference Checklist (for adults) (Williams & Shellenberger, 1996). Results of these assessments enabled students to identify their individual learning styles and sensorimotor needs for optimal learning. After receiving an orientation to materials in the sensorimotor cabinet, students were encouraged to use them in class on the basis of their individual learning style and sensorimotor needs.

Survey of Student Use of Classroom Modifications

Thirty-two students completed a written survey documenting their use of the sensorimotor materials after 40 hr of class (8 weeks, 5 hr per week). The survey gathered information on whether students used a particular item and the frequency of use during class (0–50% of the time or 50–100% of the time). Students described how using the material influenced them in class. Finally, students discussed what they liked or did not like about items in the sensorimotor cabinet and suggested changes.

Data Analysis

Inferential statistics. A repeated-measures analysis of variance for mixed design identified within-subjects differences for the various time intervals and between-subjects differences for group comparison purposes. Parametric statistics were applied because the students were randomly assigned and reflected a typical occupational therapy class (Howell, 1987; Munro, 1997). Box's Test for Equality of Covariance, Levene's Test of Equality of Variance, and Mauchly's Test of Sphericity identified whether the data met the assumptions of equality of covariance, homogeneity of variance, and compound symmetry, respectively (Munro, 1997). Post hoc pairwise comparison tests for within-subjects contrasts also identified changes within each time interval for the students as a whole group and for each of the two groups separately. Finally, regression lines were computed to predict trends in mean changes in arousal for both groups.

Descriptive statistics. The frequency and percentage of responses were collected to analyze the data from the survey that involved which sensorimotor items the students used and how frequently. In addition, traditional content analysis methods documented and analyzed narrative responses to the subjective survey questions. Summaries and frequencies of the individual student responses were reported.

Results

Within-Subjects and Between-Subjects Differences

Although Box's Test for Equality of Covariance and Levene's Test for Equality of Error Variances were not significant, the data were significant for Mauchly's Test of Sphericity. For this reason, the multivariate approach was used (Munro, 1997). Table 1 displays the results of between-subjects and within-subjects comparisons. A significant within-subjects difference was evident when comparing the levels of arousal for all of the students among the six time periods collected during the class, $F(5, 26) = 4.40$, $p = .005$. However, no significance was evident

Table 1
Results of Repeated-Measures Analysis of Variance for Ratings of Arousal During Class

Interval	Control Group[a]	Experimental Group[b]	Total
Comparison of between-group means at various intervals of class			
First hour			
1 (20 min)	7.40	6.69	7.02
2 (35 min)	7.27	6.27	6.73
3 (45 min)	6.82	6.65	6.72
Second hour[c]			
4 (15 min)	7.53	7.22	7.36
5 (30 min)	6.78	7.10	6.95
6 (45 min)	7.83	7.70	7.77
Significant pairwise comparisons for levels of arousal (p)			
2 and 6		0.015	0.006
3 and 4	0.036		0.017
3 and 6	0.005	0.019	0.048
4 and 6			0.048
5 and 6		0.030	0.000

Note. For within-subjects differences, $F = 4.40$ and $p = .005$; for between-subjects differences, $F = 1.37$ and $p = .26$. [a] $n = 16$. [b] $n = 17$. [c] A 10-min break was provided between the first and second hour.

regarding between-subjects differences, $F(5, 26) = 1.37$, $p = .26$, when comparing the students in the modified classroom with the control group. Post hoc pairwise comparisons were made of the six interval ratings of level of arousal. A significant difference was evident between intervals 2 and 6, 3 and 4, 3 and 6, 4 and 6, and 5 and 6 when analyzing data from all students. Similar within-subjects comparisons were analyzed separately for students in the modified and traditional classroom. Significant pairwise contrasts occurred between intervals 3 and 4 and 3 and 6 for the control group and between intervals 2 and 6, 3 and 6, and 5 and 6 for the experimental group. In all pairwise comparisons, the level of arousal was higher during the later time interval. Finally, the slope of the regression line was 1.38 in the modified class ($R^2 = .73$) compared with .24 for the traditional class ($R^2 = .03$), which suggests a stronger upward trend in arousal in students who used the sensorimotor materials (see Figure 1).

Descriptive Findings

Nearly all of the students (87.5%) used materials from the sensorimotor cabinet during class. When comparing use of materials in the three main sensorimotor areas of movement, touch, and objects to put into one's mouth, the highest percentage of students used items to put into one's mouth (37.5%–50%), followed by items to touch (12.5%–40.7%) and opportunities to move (12.5%–37.5%) (see Table 2). The most frequently used food items were crunchy foods such as pretzels, low-fat cereals, crackers (50%); gum (47%); and sour gummy worms (47%). When comparing the use of the touch items, the students used the Koosh balls most often (40.7%). Only four students used the Move-n-Sit cushions, and only one student consistently used a cushion. A larger percentage of students (37.5%) preferred to use the pillows at their desks. When comparing the amount of time that students used the materials during class, a higher percentage of students used the materials between 0% and 50% of the time (21.6%) versus between 50% and 100% of the time (14.0%). The items that students used most often for more than 50% of the class time were gum (eight students), pillows (seven students), and Koosh balls (six students).

Discussion

By using the Alert Program (Williams & Shellenberger, 1992) as a guide, a traditional classroom was modified by offering a cabinet filled with sensorimotor materials for second-year occupational therapy students to use in regulating levels of arousal during class and to create a less formal learning environment. An overwhelming majority of students (87.5%) used the materials and found them to be helpful either in staying alert or in providing an outlet for excess energy. After evaluating learning styles and sensorimotor preferences, students experimented with the use of sensorimotor materials in class during an 8-week period. This allowed them to identify and use the most effective sensorimotor strategies

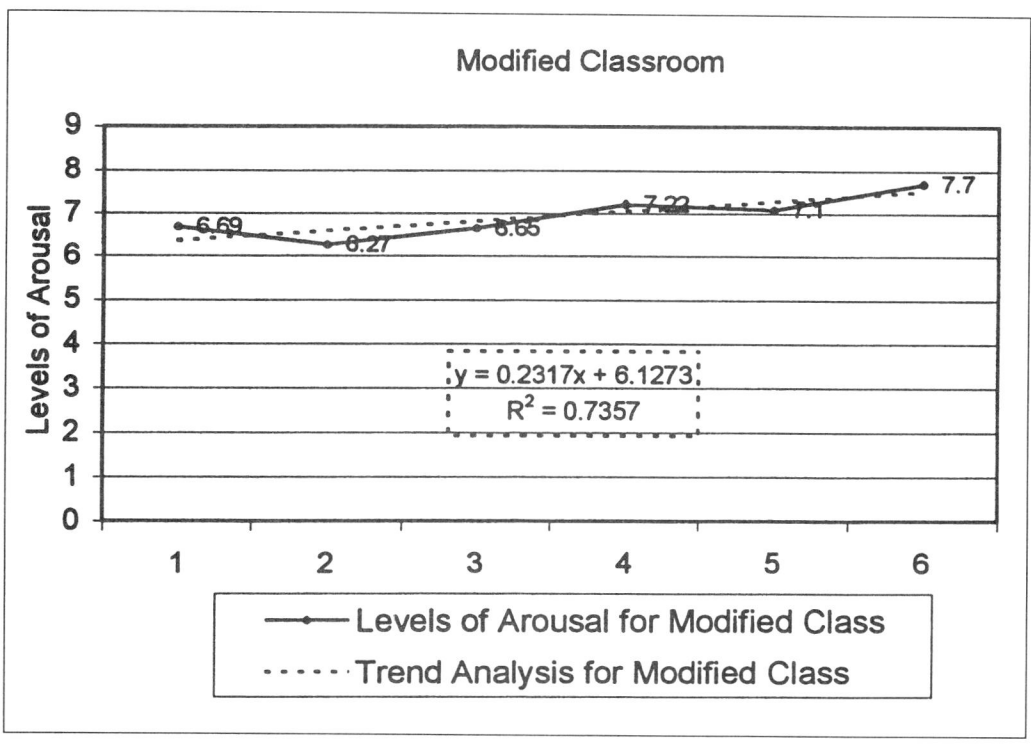

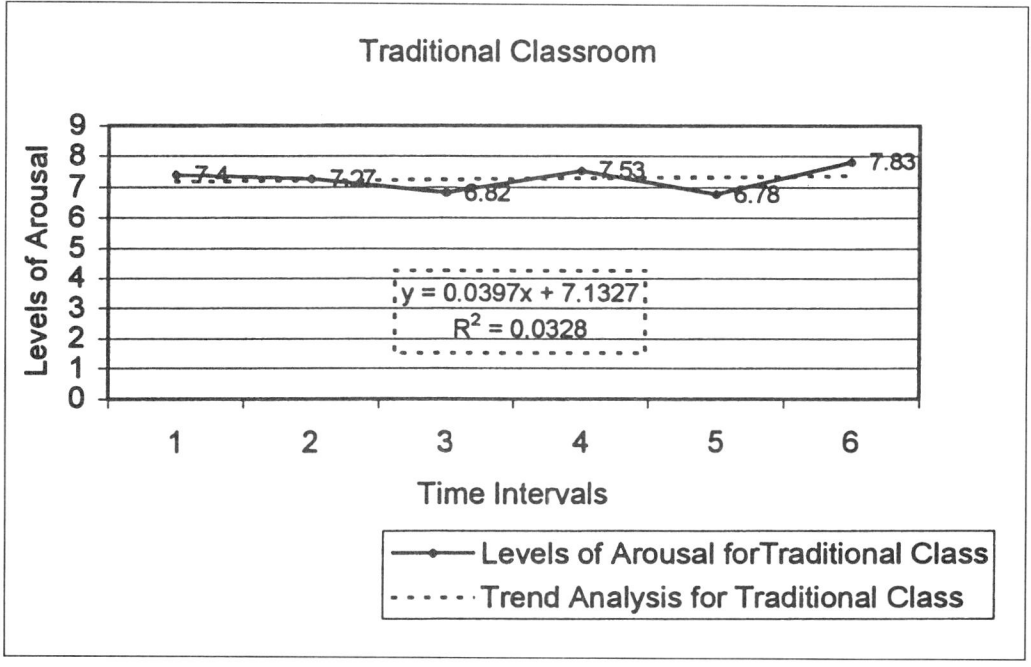

Figure 1. Graphs of trend analysis for levels of arousal in modified and traditional classrooms.

Table 2
Use of Sensorimotor Materials in the Classroom: Frequencies and Percentages

Material	Frequency of Use (%)			
	Never Used	Used Sometimes	Used 0–50% of the Time	Used 50–100% of the Time
Move				
Move-n-Sit cushions	28 (87.5)	4 (12.5)	3 (9.4)	1 (3.1)
Pillows	20 (62.5)	12 (37.5)	5 (15.6)	7 (21.9)
Touch				
Fleece blankets	29 (91.6)	0	0	3 (9.4)
Koosh balls	19 (59.4)	13 (40.7)	7 (21.9)	6 (18.8)
Spongy balls	22 (68.8)	10 (31.3)	6 (18.8)	4 (12.5)
Thera-Band tubing	28 (87.5)	4 (12.5)	3 (9.4)	1 (3.1)
Mouth				
Gum	17 (53.1)	15 (47.0)	7 (21.9)	8 (25.1)
Crunchy foods	16 (50.0)	16 (50.0)	11 (34.4)	5 (15.6)
Hard candy	19 (59.4)	13 (40.7)	8 (25.1)	5 (15.6)
Chewy candy	20 (62.5)	12 (37.5)	9 (28.2)	3 (9.4)
Sour gummy worms	17 (53.1)	15 (47.0)	10 (31.2)	5 (15.6)

Note. n = 32.

and experience firsthand their benefits on regulating arousal. The intent was for students to use this experience to improve their ability to apply the Alert Program to children in school-based practice.

By using a quasi-experimental design, a comparison of student self-ratings of arousal at six time intervals during a 2-hr class indicated no significant differences between the modified and traditional classroom. Numerous factors may have influenced these results. First, a 2-hr class period may not have been long enough to see the full effect of the modified classroom materials on student arousal. Second, student awareness of being a part of the study automatically appeared to heighten their levels of arousal. After the study, students in the control group reported that they had been unusually vigilant during class and waited to see whether a different teaching strategy would be used. This factor may explain the reason for fairly high levels of arousal at the beginning of class for the control group. Time of day may have influenced arousal as well. Initial levels of arousal were higher for the 8:00 a.m. control group than for the 10:00 a.m. experimental group. A better match may have existed between preferred learning time and class time for the control group (Dunn & Dunn, 1987).

Although no significant difference in levels of arousal was evident between the two groups, the experimental group had three significant pairwise comparisons (intervals 2 and 6, 3 and 6, and 5 and 6), with each indicating a progressive increase in arousal from the beginning to the end of class. The control group had only one significant pairwise comparison between an earlier level and the end of class (3 and 6). In addition, the slope for the modified classroom supports a stronger upward trend in arousal than in the control group. One possible explanation is that a cumulative effect may have occurred over time from using materials in the modified classroom. Another observation is that for both groups, levels of arousal increased before the 10-min break and directly before the end of class. Students' arousal levels may increase in anticipation of the end of class.

Analyzing survey results identified trends in student use of the sensorimotor materials. Of the 33 students, 29 (87.5%) chose to use materials in the sensorimotor cabinet. Overall, students enjoyed having freedom of choice regarding the use of the items and believed that having them available made the classroom less formal and added an element of novelty and fun. Students who did not use the materials indicated that they used their own strategies for regulating arousal (e.g., drinking coffee, sipping water, using a highlighter in class, wiggling their feet). Of the students who used the materials, the students used the items to put into their mouths most often, with crunchy foods, gum, and gummy worms being the most popular. Chewing provides proprioceptive input (i.e., "heavy work") to the jaw, which results in enhanced neural organization and regulation of arousal (Williams & Shellenberger, 1992). This oral-motor activity can either increase levels of arousal for a student who is losing attention or can decrease arousal during stressful situations (e.g., taking a test). A clear majority of students in this study indicated that chewing gum, crunchy foods, and candy helped them to stay alert; a few students indicated that chewing crunchy foods was calming. These results support the need for instructors to be flexible in allowing food and beverage consumption in the classroom as long as students are discrete and clean up afterward.

Students used materials that provide touch the second most frequently, with Koosh balls a clear favorite. Items offering opportunities to touch in this study all provided tactile input to the hands and fingers as well as proprioceptive input if the students pulled, squeezed, or twisted the items. Approximately half of the students indicated that manipulating these items helped them to maintain attention, whereas the other half indicated that fidgeting with the toy released excess energy and was calming. When asked what other items they fidgeted with, the students listed several objects, including paper clips, pens, binder clips, and twisting one's hair. The remaining item in the touch category, fleece blankets, was added to the sensorimotor cabinet at student request. Several students indicated that they like to study with a soft blanket or throw wrapped around their shoulders because it gave them a feeling of warmth and comfort. On the basis of this suggestion, two fleece throws were added to the sensorimotor cabinet. Being wrapped in a soft blanket provides a sense of containment and can regulate temperature for those students who typically feel cold. Students indicated that the blankets helped them feel warm, cozy, and safe. Two students suggested that more blankets be available.

The smallest number of students used materials offering opportunities to move. Only two items were available to modify movement in the classroom (Move-n-Sit cushions, pillows). The Move-n-Sit cushions allow for subtle weight shifting while sitting and a softer surface on which to sit. The four students who reported using these items indicated that the opportunity to move while sitting helped improve attending and sitting posture. This movement provides proprioceptive input to muscles and joints that helps the nervous system regulate arousal (Williams & Shellenberger, 1992). Students who chose not to use these cushions found the movement to be too distracting. Students clearly preferred the pillows versus the Move-n-Sit cushions. Most students reported that the pillows helped to improve comfort while sitting at their desks. Three students indicated that holding the pillow on their laps or leaning on it helped them to be more relaxed. Having pillows available in a traditional classroom filled with desks offers an inexpensive way in which to make the learning environment more informal for global learners.

One limitation of this pilot study is that the comparison of levels of arousal between the modified and traditional classroom resulted from only one 2-hr class period. To expand on these results, future studies must compare levels of arousal between the two groups for a longer period (e.g., several class sessions) and must use a larger pool of participants. Another limitation is that only one measure of arousal was used as baseline data for the students. For future studies, a series of baseline measures of student arousal is necessary.

Conclusions

Although the comparison of levels of arousal in the modified versus traditional classroom in this pilot study did not yield significant between-group differences, the within-interval data and slope lines suggest a positive cumulative effect from use of the sensorimotor materials during a 2-hr class. After an 8-week period of use, survey results indicated that most students used the sensorimotor materials in class, with preferences for objects to put into their mouths versus objects to touch and opportunities to move. This study supports the notion that students have individual sensorimotor preferences for regulating their arousal that a traditional classroom may not meet. Professors may need to question traditional assumptions about classroom design and furniture. This project introduces faculty members to the possibility of offering various sensorimotor materials within the classroom to support college students' individual sensorimotor needs for maintaining arousal. ■

Acknowledgment

This project was supported by a 1998 Teaching Fellowship Award from the University Center for Teaching and Learning, Cleveland State University.

References

Boulmetis, J., & Sabula, A. (1996). Achievement gains via instruction that matches learning style perceptual preferences. *Journal of Continuing Higher Education, 44,* 15–24.

Dunn, R. (1988). Capitalizing on students' perceptual strengths to ensure literacy while engaging in conventional lecture/discussion. *Reading Psychology, 9,* 431–453.

Dunn, R. (1990). Understanding the Dunn and Dunn Learning Styles Model and the need for individual diagnosis and prescription. *Reading, Writing, and Learning Disabilities, 6,* 223–247.

Dunn, R. (1991). Redesigning the conventional classroom to respond to learning style differences. *Inter-Ed., 18,* 83–87.

Dunn, K., & Dunn, R. (1987). Dispelling outmoded beliefs about student learning. *Educational Leadership, 44,* 55–62.

Dunn, R., & Dunn, K. (1991). Footloose and free to learn. *Principal, 70,* 34–37.

Dunn, R., Dunn, K., & Price, G. (1989). *Learning Style Inventory (LSI).* (Available from Price Systems, Box 1818, Lawrence, KS 66044)

Dunn, R., Griggs, S. A., Olson, J., & Beasley, M. (1995). A meta-analytic validation of the Dunn and Dunn Model of Learning Style preferences. *Journal of Educational Research, 88,* 353–362.

Dunn, R., & Nelson, B. (1996). Introducing educational administration candidates to learning-style approaches. *Educational Considerations, 24,* 44–47.

Griggs, D., Griggs, S. A., Dunn, R., & Ingham, J. (1994). Accommodating nursing students' diverse learning styles. *Nurse Educator, 19,* 41–93.

Hodges, H. (1985). An analysis of the relationships among preferences for a formal/informal design, one element of learning style, academic achievement, and attitudes of seventh and eighth grade students in remedial mathematics classes in a New York City junior high school. *Dissertation Abstracts International, 45,* 2791A.

Howell, D. C. (1987). *Statistical methods for psychology.* Boston: PWS.

Lenehan, M. C., Dunn, R., Ingham, J., Signer, B., & Murray, J. B. (1994). Effects of learning-style intervention on college students' achievement, anxiety, anger, and curiosity. *Journal of College Student Development, 35,* 461–466.

Munro, B. H. (1997). *Statistical methods for health care research.* Philadelphia: Lippincott.

Shea, T. (1983). An investigation of the relationships among preferences for the learning style element of design, selected instructional environments, and reading achievement with ninth-grade students to improve administrative determinants concerning effective educational facilities. *Dissertation Abstracts International, 44,* 2004A–2007A.

Williams, M., & Shellenberger, S. (1992). *An introduction to "How Does Your Engine Run?": The Alert Program for Self-Regulation.* Albuquerque, NM: Therapy Works.

Williams, M., & Shellenberger, S. (1996). *"How Does Your Engine Run?": A leader's guide to the Alert Program for Self-Regulation.* Albuquerque, NM: Therapy Works.

INSTRUCTIONAL METHODS

Understanding the Nature of Process

Terra Ruppert

Terra Ruppert, MS, OTR, is Director, Department of Occupational Therapy, Tomball College, Tomball, Texas, and Doctoral Student, Occupational Therapy, Texas Woman's University, Denton, Texas.

This article explores a method for teaching future occupational therapy practitioners the concept of process versus product. Emphasis was on students' understanding of the nature of process because of its dominating role in patient treatment and its ultimate effect on treatment outcomes. We measured preinstruction and postinstruction changes in overall creative potential and analyzed narrative responses to preinstruction and postinstruction experiences. Although quantitative results did not reveal major changes in creative ability, qualitative analysis yielded a richness of student understanding of the nature of process. In particular, students experienced the phenomena of risk taking; increased self-confidence; the confrontation of the fears and frustrations that accompany a new task; a greater appreciation for the concept of time; and the need to find balance in work, rest, and leisure. In addition, students were able to parallel their experiences of the challenges of the class assignment to future patients who likewise will experience new challenges through the process of treatment.

The practice of occupational therapy concerns both the *what* and *how* of performance. The *what* of performance refers to the product or outcome of therapy, and the *how* of performance refers to the process or method by which the outcome was reached. *Process* as a concept can be complex to analyze and understand because of its multifaceted and ever-dynamic components. Yet, because process is so integral to the practice of occupational therapy, the education of future occupational therapy practitioners must include a firm grasp of understanding the nature of process. This article introduces one method for teaching the nature of process. Although our institution applied the method to occupational therapy assistant students, it has broad relevance to the education of future occupational therapy practitioners at all levels.

Purpose

The Occupational Therapy Assistant Program at Tomball College in Tomball, Texas, recently enrolled students for the first time. The pioneering of a new program brings with it opportunities to try new and perhaps innovative approaches. In the first semester of the program students are involved in two courses, Introduction to Occupational Therapy and Activities and Analysis I, which are specific to the occupational therapy assistant role. The course description for Activities and Analysis I is as follows:

> An introduction to the history of activities as they relate to occupational therapy theory and practice. Through individual, dyadic, and group methods, students will analyze the components of tasks and their relation to human performance. Students will be introduced to a variety of therapeutic media and will achieve

> the basic skills of primary activities. Safe techniques for proper lifting, transportation, equipment storage, and the handling of hazardous materials as they pertain to both client and therapist will be identified. (North Harris Montgomery Community College District, 1998–1999, p. 190)

Through the analysis of activities during this course, students learn to understand that activities and tasks involve dimensions of process and product. My experience in practice has been that this concept is not always clear to even the most experienced and apparently well-trained practitioners. The concept of *product* is generally simple to discern because through the nature of the product placed before oneself; however, the concept of *process* is more difficult to grasp because of its complexities and lack of tangibility. Susan Tracy, a pioneer in occupational therapy, has been quoted as saying, "The patient is the product, not the article he makes" (as cited in Bing, 1995, p. 8).

The first objective outlined for the Activities and Analysis I course is, "Verbalize and demonstrate understanding of the difference between process and product in task performance" (Ruppert, 1998, p. 1). Thus, Tomball College has taken an innovative approach to help students accomplish this objective. In designing the approach, we considered part of the overall program philosophy. The philosophy states:

> The principles of the Occupational Adaptation frame of reference (Schkade & Schultz, 1992) are the core of this structural framework wherein occupation is characterized by active participation, meaning to the person, and the formation of a product that is the output of a process. Adaptation is identified as a change in the functional state of the person as a result of movement toward relative mastery over occupational challenges. Thus, occupational adaptation is a state of competency in occupational functioning toward which human beings aspire and is the driving force of intrinsic motivation.
>
> The holistic principles of Occupational Adaptation form a parallel process in the Occupational Therapy Assistant Program at Tomball College; wherein occupational therapy is not merely something that a therapist does to or with a patient or client but that the principles can be applied to the self. Actual understanding of the principles will come as the student applies what he or she learns to master and adapt to his or her own challenges as he or she simultaneously learn methods, principles, and skills to assist others in their adaptation process. The student develops a repertoire of experience from which to draw meaningful application of purposeful activity for a particular client. Thus, ultimately the student can apply knowledge on a continuum of wellness to illness with an understanding of the diverse nature of individuals. (Tomball College, 1998, pp. 23–24)

Therefore, to truly understand the dimensions of process, students must experience the nature of process themselves in a manner that challenges them occupationally. Similarly, another objective of the course states that students are to "experience and analyze the process of occupational challenge and task mastery" (Ruppert, 1998, p. 1). Throughout the course, students will have opportunities to engage in various unfamiliar media (e.g., clay, woodwork, leatherwork), all of which may provide some degree of occupational challenge and a generally well-defined product outcome.

In addition to these challenges, students will engage in a self-paced study of the book *Drawing on the Right Side of the Brain* (Edwards, 1989). As the syllabus states,

> Each student will develop his or her own portfolio of drawings based on the self-paced assignments in *Drawing on the Right Side of the Brain*. Portfolios will be graded on completion of all assignments. Students will present their drawings in class and will participate in a group discussion on the process and meaning of the assignments and their relationship to occupational performance. (Ruppert, 1998, p. 1)

Through engagement in the exercises outlined in the book, students will experience what Edwards (1989) called a "shift in thought and perception" (p. 4) and thus will be able to draw more realistically. The book provides numerous graphic examples of before-and-after pictures of persons who have applied this process. The examples are startling and almost unbelievable in that within a period of approximately 4 months, the artwork will have progressed from very basic and childlike drawings to professional-looking portraits. The author insisted that these persons do not suddenly become talented; rather, she concluded that they were able to "see things in a different way" (Edwards, 1989, p. 4) through a shift in their awareness and way of thinking. Edwards stated:

> Drawing, pleasurable and rewarding though it is, is but a key to open the door to other goals. My hope is that *Drawing on the Right Side of the Brain* will help you expand your powers as an individual through increased awareness of your own mind and its workings. (p. 6)

We chose this particular drawing task for students because it provides a degree of challenge great enough to tap their personal resources and can, if the process is effectively engaged, bring about a high level of success.

Method

Participants

Thirteen occupational therapy assistant students already enrolled in their first semester of academic work participated in this study. The participants ranged in age from 25 to 54 years and came from various backgrounds, including having completed a bachelor's degree to having completed no previous college course work. All participants attended the same two occupational therapy assistant courses throughout the semester (Introduction to Occupational Therapy and Activities and Analysis I). Some attended other courses simultaneously, such as freshman English, anatomy and physiology, speech, and psychology.

Procedure

Quantitative tools and qualitative methods measured the effects of this approach to help participants understand experientially the nature of process. We administered both measurements before and after application of the innovative method.

The Cree Questionnaire (Thurstone & Mellinger, 1995) is a research-based psychological test of creativity that asserts that creatively productive persons tend to differ from less creative persons. We used the test to show the relationship of the innovative method to changes in creativity. The 58-item test measures 10 dimensions of creativity that are then grouped under four broad headings:

1. *Social orientation*: dominance versus submission and independence versus conformity
2. *Work orientation*: autonomous versus structured environment and pressured versus relaxed situations
3. *Internal functioning*: high versus low energy level, fast versus slow reaction, and high versus low ideational spontaneity
4. *Interests*: high versus low theoretical interests, high versus low artistic interests, and high versus low mechanical interests

From the raw scores, we generated normalized standard scores and interpreted them in terms of low, average, or high creativity.

In addition, the participants wrote a one-page paper about their thoughts and feelings regarding their preinstruction drawings. The book had the students engage in the following four preinstruction drawings:

1. Draw a picture of someone (the head only)
2. Draw a picture of a person without looking at anyone
3. Draw a picture of your own hand
4. Draw a picture of a chair by looking at a real chair

After the participants completed the instructional portion of the book wherein they were assigned 25 drawings, they again wrote—this time a one-page to two-page paper—about their thoughts and feelings about their drawings. On completion of the project, participants displayed their before-and-after pictures to the class at a gallery showing in which they discussed their experiences and the nature of process.

Results

Although the quantitative data did not reveal notable outcomes, the qualitative data, in contrast, were rich with information.

Quantitative Data

One participant withdrew from the program before the halfway point of the semester, leaving 12 participants to review as a group and as separate entities. In analyzing the overall creative potential scores from the Cree Questionnaire, we discarded the scores of the two participants who showed no change in creativity from the preinstruction to the postinstruction test. A Wilcoxon signed rank test (T) was used to evaluate the data because it requires fewer assumptions than a paired t test. No significant increase in creativity scores was revealed after the innovative method ($T = 22.5$, $p < 0.05$; ranks for increases totaling 22.5, and ranks for decreases totaling 32.5).

Qualitative Data

The following excerpts are from the prenarrative and postnarrative portions of the participants' writings on the process of engaging in the assigned task. Some samples of drawings displayed at the gallery showing are provided.

Student A: Postnarrative: "At times the project seemed tedious. (I was probably distracted with the thought of my test next week!) At this point I realized that when patients are worried about their health, finances, or family affairs, it can affect their production and how they view the task assigned to them as well."

Student B: Prenarrative: "It is a wonderful feeling to have permission to take the time to be creative" (see Figure 1). Postnarrative: "I experienced many feelings along the process of this assignment. I found that when doing something creative, that I really needed to be in the right frame of mind to draw. Sometimes I had time, but just did not feel like drawing" (see Figure 2).

Student C: Prenarrative: "It was not easy, but once I cleared my mind of the 'can't do it' with 'do your best,' I began drawing." Postnarrative: "In the beginning, my confidence was weak. My skills and abilities in creating a picture were underdeveloped. I did not believe in myself….Shifting to a particular way of seeing, after understanding what I read, I viewed my drawings differently, and they began to look better."

Student D: Prenarrative: "Doing this exercise was very scary for me. I never considered myself very good at art of any kind. As I was drawing, I felt such a feeling of inadequacy. You are wishing you could do better, but any attempts to improve your work are futile" (see Figure 3). Postnarrative: "Now I have learned to look at objects differently. My initial thoughts were that this was going to be really hard and it was….I do not feel scared to draw now….I have more confi-

Instructional Methods

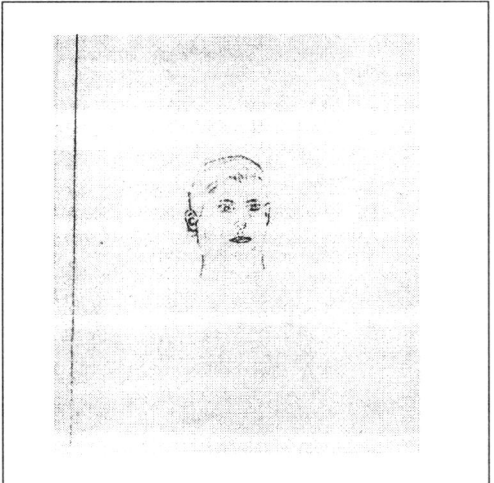

Figure 1. Student B: preinstruction drawing.

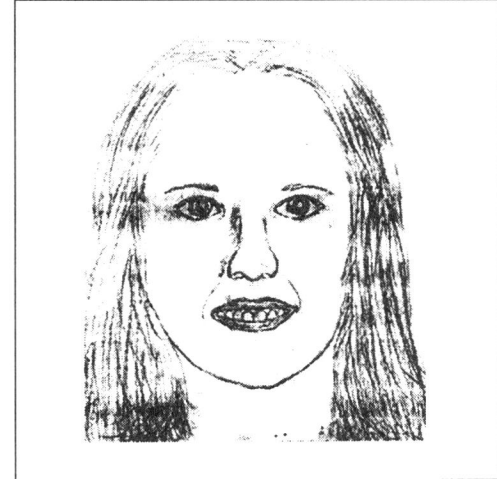

Figure 2. Student B: postinstruction drawing.

dence in my abilities now....It was an extremely difficult project, but I benefited in many ways. Some I'm sure I have yet to realize. It was a good exercise in time management, coping skills, and self-control" (see Figure 4).

Student E: Postnarrative: "I felt really guilty for doing the drawing when I knew that there was homework to do. I kept putting my drawings off until I had more time, but I never ended up with more time. I really ended up with less time to do them" (see Figures 5 and 6).

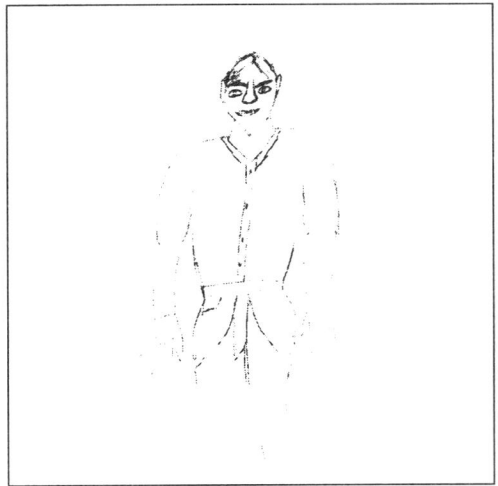

Figure 3. Student D: preinstruction drawing.

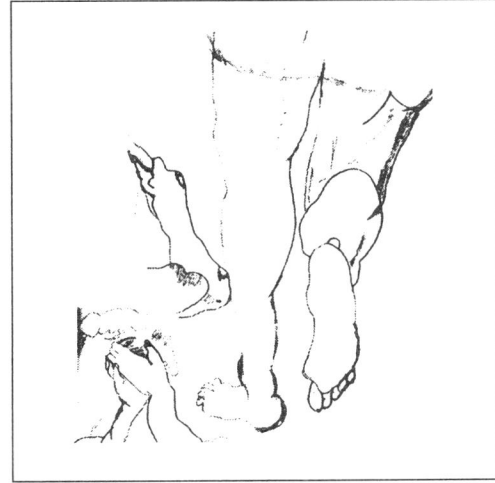

Figure 4. Student D: postinstruction drawing.

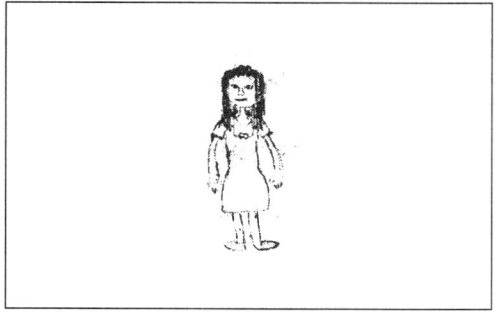 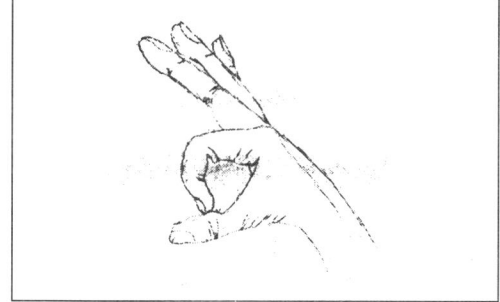

Figure 5. Student E: preinstruction drawing.   **Figure 6.** Student E: postinstruction drawing.

Student H: Prenarrative: "As an adult, I am expected to behave and think like one, but my drawing would not be comparable to an adult's work, and that was the scary part." Postnarrative: "In my preinstruction drawings, I didn't see the objects in their whole forms. But in the postinstruction drawings, I had to pause, look at the object for some time, and, if possible, draw the shape. As I moved on with my drawings and became fully engrossed, I felt relaxed and was oblivious to the world around me....It felt so good to become one with the drawing. It has increased my confidence to try and dabble in other areas of art to see what I can learn from those areas so that I become more insightful and analytical in areas of my life. In the field of occupational therapy, one needs to be very open-minded and try to see things from the client's perspective so that one can initiate the appropriate treatments. When practitioners see things in their totality, they are also able to discern underlying concerns and find possible creative solutions to patients' problems. When we see things in totality and not in pieces, we enforce the use of the holistic approach."

Student I: Postnarrative: "Looking back through my artwork, I am reminded of the various processes that I had to go through. Some were very rewarding, and a few were frustrating....I saw amazing similarities in this [drawing three objects of the same size from different perspectives] and how we need to deal with our patients. Everyone is different, and although they might have similar problems, you should never compare them or try to put them in the same category."

Student J: Postnarrative: "In both sets of drawings I had major problems in suffering from anxieties. Time management was an issue in doing both sets of my drawings. I put this assignment off until just days of the due date. I attempted twice to spend time working on the project, but I always made it last after other studies. Finally, the last week...I had nine drawings left to draw....I never felt mastery on any level of the assignment."

Student K: Prenarrative: "When I first started to draw the pictures, the drawing tired me visually and took a lot of effort and time" (see Figure 7). Postnarrative: "I have taken the risk and delved into something I had thought I had no talent for at all. Someone once said that beautiful things—music, art, friendship—are what make life worth living. As a [future] COTA, I want to convey to my patients that I have experienced the apprehension and doubt in myself to attempt something new. I want them to realize that going through the process is what is therapeutic, that the product is their expression" (see Figure 8).

Student L: Postnarrative: "It was very difficult to find the time to sit for half an hour or more at a time....I thought it would be a great stress reliever. I sure was wrong. I struggled a lot with beginning my drawings. Sometimes it would take me a half an hour just to start" (see Figures 9 and 10).

Student M: Prenarrative: "I realized that even making the simple face, person, chair, and hand was a difficult task." Postnarrative: "I am amazed how my perception of my environment has changed after doing my drawings....Noticing what is really before you is a wonderful way to see the world."

Discussion

The lack of significance in the results of the Cree Questionnaire may be because of the small sample size ($n = 12$). A pooling of the data from future classes may alleviate this limitation. However, in examining preinstruction and postinstruction scores on the Cree Questionnaire, along with the drawings and narrative responses for each participant, some interesting findings are evident.

In one of the subtests involving self-confidence (dominance vs. submission), 8 participants showed an increase from preinstruction to postinstruction scores. This is evident when looking at their preinstruction and postinstruction drawings in which a marked difference is evident in the size of the objects drawn. Before receiving instructions, students produced small and often light drawings in the middle of the page. Drawings completed near the end of the instructional period

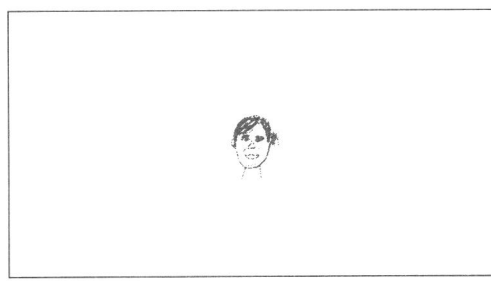

Figure 7. Student K: preinstruction drawing.

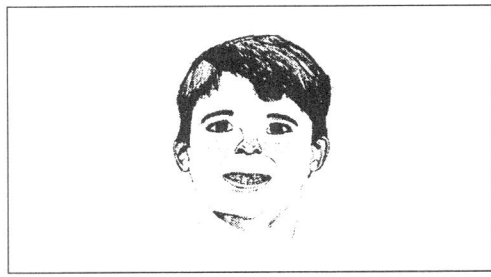

Figure 8. Student K: postinstruction drawing.

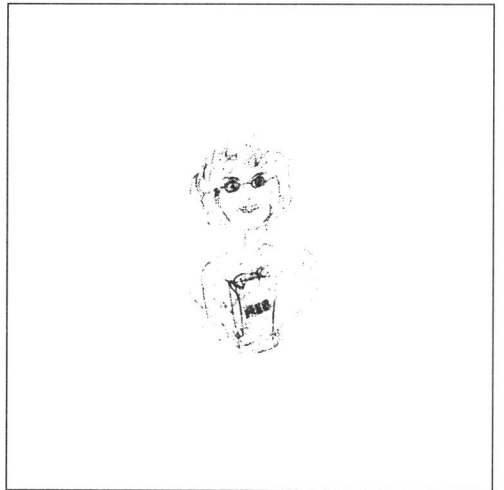 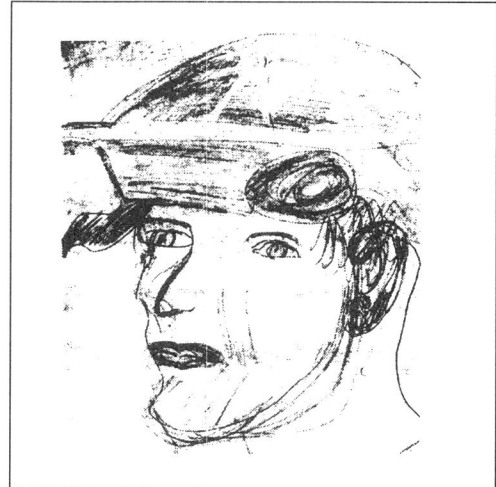

Figure 9. Student L: preinstruction drawing. **Figure 10.** Student L: postinstruction drawing.

almost filled the page and were much darker. No longer were the participants making lightly penciled, small, seemingly hesitant drawings. The postinstruction drawings display a bolder and more self-confident approach. Through their product, participants seem to be expressing the process of an increase in self-confidence over time as well as an increase in risk taking.

The shift from the use of the "left brain" to the "right brain" is a nontemporal process, and interestingly, this process is an area where several students struggled. Time became an important element, and participants discussed this in terms of needing "permission"; "looking for time"; "having difficulty focusing time"; and, more generally, time management. One participant was able to say that he felt "oblivious to time." On the Cree Questionnaire, Students B and E showed an increase in the high versus low energy subtest that is indicative of an abundance of energy and general haste and impatience (Thurstone & Mellinger, 1995). They also mentioned having difficulty dealing with time as they engaged in the task. Conversely, Students C, F, I, and K showed an increase on the Cree Questionnaire in their ability to work better under pressure and did not mention time as a factor in their narratives. Student J reported waiting until the last minute to work on the task and sensed numerous anxieties because of this. She expressed an overall dissatisfaction with the task and an increase in creativity in only one area on the Cree Questionnaire. Thus, she did not give herself time to engage in the process of the task, and she did not give the task the full merit of the time required. Ultimately, as a result, her understanding of process was thwarted. Likewise, patients may procrastinate on projects where they fear they may fail or at least may experience as unpleasant. Often such a patient will minimally engage in the task, will not perform adequately as a result, and then will later count the task as one that was not useful. Even though a task may have all the earmarks of success as defined by the occupational therapy practitioner (e.g., meaning, purpose, motivational intent), the emotional content associated with a task may delay engagement. As a result, time becomes no longer a friend, but a foe.

During the gallery showing in class, participants displayed a preinstruction and a postinstruction drawings and talked about the processes that they experienced. For the most part, they verbalized what they had written in their narrative formats. However, a few expressed that they would have liked to have had the author of *Drawing on the Right Side of the Brain* present to coach them when they started to drift from the correct methods. This idea led to a more focused discussion about the role that the occupational therapy practitioner plays in guiding a patient through his or her own process of recovery and change. Many participants expressed an increased understanding for metaphorical relationships, particularly as they pertain to their future roles in working with patients. In particular, the occupational therapy practitioner's roles may include guide, prompter, educator, advisor, cheerleader, and so forth. The question that surfaces is: At what point does the practitioner shift roles in such a way as to allow room for patient risk taking that would lead to greater patient self-accomplishment and, ultimately, greater patient independence?

As the last participant to show her drawings to the class (and seemingly the most reluctant), Student J verbalized an increase in overall understanding about process once she began to reflect on the statements that the others made during the class discussion. She expressed an awareness of having limited experiences in her life and of being reluctant and fearful to engage in anything new that would take her out of her comfort zone. Many participants verbalized embarrassment at showing their drawings to the class but went on to display numerous drawings, even though only two were required. This phenomenon may be because of the increase in self-confidence as discussed earlier and may be reflective of an underlying sense of pride in their accomplishments that they may not feel comfortable admitting verbally to the other class members. Similarly, patients may verbalize feelings of embarrassment or inadequacy, yet their performance, in contrast, demonstrates the pride of accomplishment.

One of the most surprising outcomes was the participants' awareness of how difficult balancing work, rest, and leisure can be. Most put the task, which was a homework assignment to be graded, in the leisure category. At several points throughout the semester, the participants verbalized guilt for using time to do the drawings because they were "supposed to be fun." In their narratives, several participants verbalized feeling as though they should accomplish all of their "work" tasks first (e.g., studying anatomy) before sitting down to draw. In essence, they seemed to be saying to themselves that taking time out to do something enjoyable is not acceptable. Likewise, patients do not always take seriously tasks that are embedded in elements of "fun."

Most remarkable were the participants' abilities to generalize their experiences gained from this challenge to the possible experiences and challenges that their future patients will face. They were able to express an understanding of the self-doubts and personal fears that accompany embarking on uncharted territory. Likewise, they were able to experience and understand the frustrations that coincide with their own perceived lack of success in performance and a fear of scrutiny by others regarding task performance. As such, they were able to compare these personal insights to the experiences of a patient who may have a particular trauma or disability and may be expected to achieve a certain level of performance regarding the task or challenges that the occupational therapy practitioner provides. In essence, the participants had to confront fears about their own performance and work through them. As a result, those who took on the challenge came out victorious and strengthened. The assigned task or challenge for a patient and a student may be different, but much of the process is similar.

Conclusion

Engaging in process is one thing; acknowledging process is another; and understanding process is yet something else altogether. Within this group of students were varying levels of knowledge regarding process. Students who invested time in the process of drawing seemed to learn the most about the nature of process in general. These are the students who seemed to understand that this particular task was not about drawing but about self-growth and generalizing self-experience to situations with others outside of the self, such as patients.

Time, in relation to this study, turned out to be an important factor. Even though we all are allotted 24 hours in a day, time is a factor of relevance, and everyone experiences time differently. Inherent to the nature of process is the concept of time. Engaging in a process takes time. The nature of product, in contrast, may take little more than a momentary glance to comprehend.

Process, in relation to this task, involved challenges, risk taking, effort, and acknowledgment of feelings. Process is the place in which a person experiences purpose and meaning in occupation. Many of the students took a firm grasp of the task, found purpose and meaning in it, and were able to relate their experiences from beyond the moment to where they might understand another person's challenges, fears, and triumphs.

Like air, process is somewhat of an elusive subject. It is all around us, and we cannot live without it, yet we cannot put it in our hands. We can read about process, and we can talk about process, but we must experience process to truly understand it. This understanding of the nature of process is highly relevant to the development of effective occupational therapy practitioners because it is through process that the products of performance and function come forth. Too often as practitioners we focus on outcomes without giving reverence to the process that precedes the outcome.

Teaching an abstract concept such as process can provide its own challenges to the educator of future occupational therapy practitioners. Again, the educator may choose to discuss the concept or may choose to have students read about the concept; however, not until students experience the concept for themselves will the nature of the concept firmly take hold. Thus, engaging students in the challenges of *Drawing on the Right Side of the Brain* appears to be a most valuable tool in helping students understand the nature of process. ■

References

Bing, R. (1995). In S. Ryan (Ed.), *The certified occupational therapy assistant: Principles, concepts and techniques* (pp. 3–20). Thorofare, NJ: Slack.

Edwards, B. (1989). *Drawing on the right side of the brain.* Los Angeles: Jeremy P. Tarcher.

North Harris Montgomery Community College District. (1998–1999). *North Harris Montgomery Community College District catalog.* Houston, TX: Author.

Ruppert, T. (1998). *Activities and analysis I* [Course syllabus]. Tomball, TX: Tomball College.

Schkade, J., & Schultz, S. (1992). Occupational adaptation: Toward a holistic approach for contemporary practice. *American Journal of Occupational Therapy, 46,* 829–837.

Thurstone, T., & Mellinger, J. (1995). *Cree Questionnaire.* Rosemont, IL: NCS.

Tomball College. (1998). *Occupational therapy assistant program development plan.* Tomball, TX: Author.

INSTRUCTIONAL METHODS

Developing a Language for Discussing Writing: Composition in Occupational Therapy?

Jane Detweiler
Claudia Peyton

Jane Detweiler, PhD, is Assistant Professor, Department of English, University of Nevada, Reno, Nevada.

Claudia Peyton, PhD(c), FAOTA, is Associate Professor and Chair, Division of Occupational Therapy, University of Alabama, Birmingham, Alabama.

In recent years, occupational therapy has undergone substantial changes as its practitioners have continued to develop new conceptions of their profession along with new theoretical and methodological world views. Like many other emerging or transforming fields, occupational therapy has begun to reinvent itself as a discipline among other disciplines, a territory with a history of shifting boundaries that is changing in its relationship to other intellectual landscapes marked out by communities of academic and professional endeavor (Quiroga, 1995). Along with these disciplinary shifts, many transformations of health care and public policy have placed occupational therapists in different clinical worlds of work. In response to various intellectual, political, or economic changes, programs educating new professionals for the field have been restructuring degree programs and making decisions regarding how to teach the philosophical and practical underpinnings of the field. In current debates that center on academic versus professional school "homes" for occupational therapy programs, and on the entry-level master's degree versus the entry-level clinical doctorate, occupational therapists are reenvisioning the terrain of professional roles that clinicians may eventually fill (Pierce & Peyton, 1999).

One particularly important role for future occupational therapists, that of the occupational therapist as a writing professional, has at this point received relatively little attention in the field's reflections. Yet, in this role, many occupational therapists have made their cases for change in theories, methods, public policies, and reimbursement for services. As educators in this health discipline note the power that strong writing abilities can have for professionals, they likewise note that students seem to need increasingly more assistance in building those abilities. Occupational therapy faculty members often wonder, because students are required to take general composition courses, why these novices are not already prepared for any and all writing that they will do in their professional education. The fact that many occupational therapy students are not writing as well or as confidently as faculty members would suggest that general composition courses are not fully preparing students for the kinds of writing that health professionals need to do. Indeed, as "introductions" to college writing, these courses were never intended to acquaint every student fully with the kinds of writing expected in every discipline. Nor do most writing teachers, who are usually affiliated with an English department, necessarily know the "ins and outs" of every discipline's preferred formats, methods of citation, or situations in which writing is used. Recent research on effective writing pedagogy suggests that members of a discipline are actually best able to teach their students *how* to write at the same time that they teach *what* to write, which is the content or knowledge that the field expects new professionals to learn (Bartholomae, 1985; Bazerman, 1998; Bazerman & Paradis, 1991; Berkenkotter & Huckin, 1995; Bizzell, 1982; Brodkey, 1987; Herrington, 1985; Herrington & Moran, 1992; Prior, 1991, 1995).

If occupational therapy faculty members are best able to teach their students how to "write like an OT," then they inevitably face many curriculum design challenges. Occupational therapy programs must find answers to some key questions. Because occupational therapy faculty members are varied in their theoretical and practical backgrounds, they are likely to vary in their experience with writing and writing pedagogy. How can a program accommodate these differences? How can students learn to practice writing as effectively as they do other forms of professional practice? With all of the other aspects of curriculum that programs must address, how can faculty members set aside time for teaching writing? We have no easy answers to these questions.

However, there are some ways to begin thinking and talking about the writing that occupational therapists ask their students to do. We will discuss some strategies not only for integrating writing instruction into an existing curriculum, but also for making that writing work for teaching occupational therapy content. We will point out places to begin the work of "developing a language" for discussing the writing abilities necessary in the new professional visions of occupational therapy as a field. Ultimately, curriculum design issues are linked to the roles that a practitioner should be prepared to fill and to the nature of the profession's enterprise in the broader community of other health care professionals. As with any other curricular content, how a program views student writing will depend on how each faculty member's experience, visions of professionalism, and sense of the field's future converge in a pattern of expectations.

In three major sections, we address developing a language for discussing writing, designing a writing course, and teaching (with) writing in the field. In these sections, we move from theorizing to particularized description, from practical recommendations to providing teaching hints toward the end of the essay. After making our suggestions, we close with some final comments that are points of departure for future conversations about the role of writing in the profession of occupational therapy.

Developing a Language for Discussing Writing

For a moment, consider the diversity of theoretical, methodological, and pedagogical commitments that the various members of the faculty bring to undergraduate and graduate professional education in any particular department. This variety of commitments, when brought to bear in the collaborations involved in ongoing program design efforts, provides lively and quite productive intellectual interaction. Next, consider various educational experiences that mark the personal history of each faculty member: the sheer accumulation of knowledge, learning styles, remembered approaches to both studying and teaching, and preferences for particular structuring of classroom activities or degree programs. In any one program, the range of degrees and amounts of clinical experience may further complicate any theoretical or methodological differences, and all of these differences among faculty members can involve rather divergent experiences with and attitudes toward any professional practice. With all of these considerations in mind, imagine the variety of (usually unexamined) understandings of the writing that may take place in therapists' education or in their actual work-site activities. As occupational therapy further defines itself, teaching may be more effective when faculty members begin to develop a language (a set of theorized terms) for discussing the kinds of writing that they are asking students to do in particular courses and programs.

In a fundamental sense, developing such a language for discussing writing is similar to the many other curriculum development processes that occupational therapy educators undertake as they seek to translate the *Essentials and Guidelines for an Accredited Program for the Occupational Therapist* (American Occupational Therapy Association [AOTA]/Accreditation Council for Occupational Therapy Education [ACOTE], 1995) into a well-theorized, integrated program of studies for their students. The *Essentials and Guidelines* represent the baseline standards for educating the entry-level practitioner and serve as the basis for program reviews, although these reviews do take into account some programmatic variations (e.g., regional culture, institutional mission or philosophy, resource allocation). According to these guidelines for accreditation, occupational therapy faculty members must consider how their particular program's planning and implementation

> 1) Reflect the mission of the occupational therapy program and of the institution; 2) Identify educational goals of the program that are consistent with its mission and philosophy statements; [and] 3) Describe the set of organizing ideas that explain selection of the content, scope, and sequencing of courses. (AOTA, 1995, p. 6)

With this conceptual framework in mind, these educators then must carefully translate their program's principles into many pedagogical decisions about the appropriate kinds and sequences of learning experiences in which their students will engage (AOTA/ACOTE, 1995). Just as a program's teachers must systematically set out the details of syllabi, course objectives and content, instructional methods, and means of evaluation, we suggest that faculty members may likewise set out when and how to integrate writing into their curricular design.

Although no explicit accreditation guidelines exist that teaching writing per se should enter into such discussions and planning activities, occupational therapy educators have responded to the *Essentials and Guidelines* by systematically and creatively reflecting on their teaching practice and then putting this reflection into considered, comprehensively planned programmatic action. We invite occupational therapy faculty members to reflect creatively on integrating writing-as-pedagogy throughout their curricula and to consider thoughtfully how to use writing in a program to accomplish the goals articulated in the accreditation guidelines. For example, because writing is a symbolic, reflective activity, it is at once a mode of critical thinking or problem solving and the medium in which that thinking is communicated to others. To put this in terms of the *Essentials* for fieldwork, writing should be integrated into various efforts to promote clinical reasoning and reflective practice because the practice of writing can afford students an opportunity to conceptualize their experience and their ethical reasoning and then to convey their reflections to faculty members or preceptors (AOTA/ACOTE, 1995). Once a student performs a particular kind of intellectual activity in writing, the text is available for faculty members to evaluate in accordance with the guidelines' emphasis on systematic and continuing evaluation of student performance (AOTA/ACOTE, 1995). More importantly, we believe that the renaissance of occupation as an organizing construct for both the clinical and the didactic components of occupational therapy education is vital to the profession's future. We can establish essential connections between occupation and health through writing experiences designed for the clinical as well as the didactic portions of a curriculum, with course assignments integrated throughout the curriculum that emphasize writing as a way of learning, as a way of entering the profession, and as a way of demonstrating proficiency.

To begin developing a language for discussing writing, carefully examining how the writing each teacher currently requires of students is connected to his or her teaching philosophy, to the learning objectives of the course, to the goals of the program, and to the endeavors of the occupational therapy profession as a whole is helpful. All of these levels of conceptualization contribute to that teacher's "pedagogical world view." In composition studies (the home discipline of one coauthor of this article), classroom research has indicated that keeping in mind how writing assignments can imply, are guided by, and eventually maintain pedagogical world views is helpful (because people tend to practice as they were taught). In a recent qualitative study of writing in one occupational therapy graduate program, Detweiler (unpublished observations) found that a few key pedagogical world views were evident that underpinned the kinds of writing assigned in this program (see Table 1). In each category, we describe some of the assumptions that warrant particular teaching approaches in the classroom. The purposes that writing served in various faculty members' classrooms tended to fall into one of these tentative categories. However, areas of overlap often occurred (e.g., a teacher's emphasis changed during the course of a semester, or a particular assignment seemed to serve more than one purpose). (See Table 2 for a list of written forms used in the program's teaching that are divided into the three categories.) For our purposes, we

Table 1
Assumptions of Pedagogical World Views

World View	Assumptions
Writing to learn	■ That learning, even in professional education, is an exploratory, creative, inquiry-based process in which students must craft their own versions of the field's conventional ways of thinking and knowing.
	■ That classroom activities that are student centered and encourage a sense of student "ownership" of learning and critical thinking (i.e., focused on or deeply grounded in student interests, motivations, learning styles, and so forth rather then wholly on the teacher's preselected interests and directions) and promote learning.
	■ That learning is best evaluated individually and holistically (e.g., by considering all of the student's work during a period or progress over time).
	■ That both formal teacher-directed and informal student-directed writing exercises (and other classroom activities) can effectively produce and provide evidence of learning.
Writing to enter the profession	■ That learning in professional education is a process of internalizing particular conventions and habits of thinking (e.g., commonly accepted ways of problem solving, writing, and acting and shared assumptions about what is best and most effective practice).
	■ That classroom activities that involve the field-specific knowledge of practices in which the teacher has experience and can mentor students promote learning.
	■ That learning is best evaluated with reference to shared standards.
	■ That formal teacher-directed kinds of writing (and other classroom activities) produce better learning and evidence of learning than informal student-directed projects.
Writing to demonstrate proficiency	■ That learning in professional education is a process of acquiring a particular base of knowledge.
	■ That classroom activities that involve the field-specific knowledge or practices in which the teacher has experience and can mentor students promote learning.
	■ That learning must be evaluated with reference to shared standards, and these are profoundly tied to some shared understanding of what many or all similar students should be able to do given the constraints of a particular course or project.
	■ That formal teacher-directed kinds of writing (and other classroom activities) are the primary or only valid measure of learning.

Table 2
Writing Assignments Associated With Pedagogical World Views

World View	Writing Assignments
Writing to learn	Peer response groups
	Collaborative projects
	Short exploratory papers
	Reflective essays
	Personal (informal) journal writing
	Semester portfolios of writing
	Personal inventories
	Movie reviews and personal responses
	Web media (bulletin boards, chat rooms)
Writing to enter the profession	Article reviews
	Bibliographic papers
	Teaching modules
	Proposals (policy, research, planning)
	Assessment critiques
	Historical and theoretical papers
	Summaries
	Oral presentations of research or teaching modules
	Synthesis papers
	Teaching philosophy statements
	Case analysis and clinical case studies
	Field notes
Writing to demonstrate proficiency	Examinations
	Quizzes

refer to these tentative categories as *writing to learn,*[1] *writing to enter the profession,*[2] and *writing to demonstrate proficiency.*[3] We hope that these are useful starter terms for other occupational therapy faculty members to use as they develop a language for talking about the writing involved in various educational programs. As we have noted, although a writing assignment may operate from or incor-

---

[1]*Writing to learn* is a term and world view quite familiar to composition specialists and is a good descriptor for some of the teaching in an occupational therapy program (Berthoff, 1981; Elbow, 1973, 1981; Emig,

porate some blend of one or more of these orientations, more often than not one was dominant and guided the assignment, the classroom activities in support of the assignment, and the evaluation of the writing students produced.

With these findings in mind, we suggest the following ways to develop a language for discussing writing for faculty members in other occupational therapy programs, should they decide to revise the writing components of their teaching efforts.

1. Consider the writing assignments for each class in terms of the pedagogical orientations discussed previously, or develop some other similar way of discussing the functions that writing serves in the program's efforts. Faculty members may decide to apply writing in various ways at various points in the students' progress through the program.

2. Discuss, as a group, how each teacher's writing assignment relates to the learning objectives of the course and the program overall. If faculty members are discussing including a writing course in the program, then having faculty members discuss in detail what sorts of writing students should be doing, what sorts of writing students may do later in their careers, and how this writing relates to other ways of thinking and acting that faculty members consider important is even more crucial.

3. Clarify for students what function a given writing assignment is to serve (e.g., "This is a writing-to-learn type assignment designed to help you understand how you understand this theory," or "This writing is to focus your attention on particular stylistic requirements of this journal to help you learn to write for publication"). Herrington (1985) found that the most successful writing assignments were those that were most distinctly defined (in the written assignment and in class discussion) as either "personal learning centered" or "simulated professional situations"; in this study, "success" was described in terms of students' sense of their ability to accomplish the writ-

---

1981; Macrorie, 1970). This teaching orientation holds learning to be a highly personalized, student-centered process. Rather than simply acquiring a sort of acontextual, foundational body of facts, a student uses writing to acquire a set of critical thinking and creative skills, and this takes place in a classroom environment that encourages the student to develop a sense of personal investment in knowing. Students can learn from each other as well as from the teacher; hence, collaborative activities are involved.

[2]*Writing to enter the profession* is a world view distinct from writing to learn in that the former orientation tends to emphasize the student's passage into a professional community (Bartholomae, 1985; Bazerman, 1998; Bazerman & Paradis, 1991; Berkenkotter & Huckin, 1995; Bizzell, 1982; Brodkey, 1987; Herrington, 1985; Herrington & Moran, 1992; Prior, 1991, 1995). Teaching from this perspective involves providing an opportunity for students to analyze and to practice writing to the community's shared conventions (e.g., writing articles for professional journals).

[3]*Writing to demonstrate proficiency* reflects writing's evaluation function in pedagogy. When operating from this orientation, faculty members uphold what they consider to be universal standards of student performance as these standards manifest themselves in particular course work. The teacher links a specific classroom choice or evaluative stance to some more "global" or "objective" notion of what students should be able to do, given a sort of baseline competence and a sincere effort to learn in the course.

ing task and evaluators' understanding of what the students were to have accomplished. The latter is a particularly important consideration if faculty members not directly responsible for teaching the course or mentoring the student will be evaluating that student's writing.

4. Integrate the purposes of later, more major projects into earlier, more minor projects. In other words, if final "certifying" projects are to serve particular purposes and if faculty members want students to do particular kinds of writing, then critically reading and practicing those kinds of writing at many points (in smaller-scale efforts) throughout the program will be helpful. Furthermore, straightforwardly discussing how specific classroom efforts are related to later, more major projects will likewise be helpful.

5. Bring to attention the many forms that professional occupational therapy writing can take in various courses, and "archive" what faculty members consider to be good examples of each form (including student work) for students to examine. The former effort need not be time and energy intensive: The exercise may involve taking a few minutes in a class discussion to examine not only what the writer of a course reading is saying, but also how he or she is saying it; how the writer's argument or description is "put together"; and why the teacher, as a professional in the field, believes it is a compelling example of the writing that an occupational therapist may do. The latter effort can be a matter of finding file cabinet space, collecting faculty members' or fieldwork educators' samples or models of good document design, and establishing a procedure that ensures that students will have equal access to the archived materials (e.g., a type of library approach, with sign-out and sign-in sheets; an honor system for returning materials; a reserve policy of some kind).

6. Model critical, *rhetorical* reading as a type of critical thinking like the other problem-solving processes that the curriculum may already involve. As in the fifth suggestion, provide opportunities for students to discuss how to write for this assignment. This will be helpful when students can make connections among the writing they are required to do, other writing that they have discussed in class, and other professional writing that will be necessary in fieldwork settings. More importantly, this exercise will help students to learn another mode of interpretation that will complement the other habits of clinical interpretation that they will use in the future. Again, this exercise does not need to take a great deal of time away from other class activities. The exercise may take as little as a few minutes of group work, with a bit of small group discussion focused on the assignment prompted by, "Tell me what this assignment is asking you to do."

7. Discuss with students successful examples of the kinds of "major projects" that faculty members in the program will ultimately ask of them: Why was this sample project a good response to the specific purposes that the student and his or her advisors developed? How did this writer's approach suit his or

her future career interests (e.g., he or she wants an academic position, so this publishable article was a good choice, or he or she wants an administrative position, so that essay examining policy matters was a good choice)? Again, this activity may involve archiving good examples of student work.

8. Develop a workshop for academic and clinical educators in which these faculty members discuss the writing pedagogy in the curriculum. This workshop is one way to fulfill the ACOTE guidelines regarding communicating curricular design and instructional approaches to clinical educators who will provide fieldwork experiences for occupational therapy students. As a way of sharing information about the curriculum, academic and clinical educators may be invited to discuss (and even practice) the various kinds of writing integrated into the curriculum, how they can use it for instruction and evaluation, what various faculty members expect from student writers, and so forth.

Designing a Writing Component

We directed these comments and recommendations toward occupational therapy faculty readers and clinical faculty readers who are looking for ways to integrate writing into an existing curricular structure. Perhaps faculty members in a program have discussed including a writing course in the program. For that audience, we have prepared some other, more focused suggestions on the basis of research into writing in one occupational therapy program.

1. Never assume that the writing course will "do it all" any more than any other single course can thoroughly teach complex thought processes that professionals will need to use. Think of the writing course as an opportunity for intensive practice in the kinds of writing that students will be learning in other courses and in fieldwork experiences. In our view, this intensive practice complements, rather than replaces, the highly contextualized discussion of writing that can take place in other courses and involves a great range of topics.

2. Consider the following starter list of design options:

   - A "rhetorical analysis" element that encourages students to learn how to read critically various forms that are in use locally or in the field (e.g., research study proposals, policy statements, editorials, research reports, advocacy writing).

   - A "project development" element that can emphasize ways that students can use the writing process to create approaches, to record impressions, and to report findings of any kind. In other words, the writing course can make students aware that composing informally but systematically (e.g., brainstorming, journaling, drafting) can help ease the production of final versions of major projects.

   - A "professional experiences with the writing" element in which faculty and clinical faculty members other than occupational therapists can discuss their writing experiences and writing processes. These discussions can demystify professional writing (i.e., make it more immediately practical and concrete for students).

- A "stylistic requirements" component in which students learn how to format a piece of writing for one of the field's professional publications. This component would probably be most effective in focusing on the process of writing and revising an article for that outlet. Other options include reviewing several years' worth of a journal's publications to get a sense of what the journal considers "publishable" or collecting and reviewing several publications' submission format requirements.

3. Consider your discussions about the functions that writing serves or can serve in your program (see "Developing a Language for Discussing Writing"). Having engaged in this discussion will help faculty members design and teach the writing course or will assist whoever the program hires to design and teach it. Program faculty members will be able to specify in some detail what they want writing to do in the program, how students should be able to write, what sorts of forms are important, and what the writing expectations will be in Level I and II fieldwork components of the curriculum.

4. If the occupational therapy program hires a non–occupational therapy faculty member to teach the writing course, consider engaging a writing specialist who is interested in such concepts as writing across the curriculum or writing in the disciplines. Such a person is likely to be sensitive to your department's needs. Ask to see several examples of this person's course syllabi and writing assignments. Consider what sorts of pedagogical values these items reflect and how these values support the values in the occupational therapy curriculum design, just as department faculty members will have done with their own teaching. In designing a writing course, faculty members may also consider the following teaching options:

- A "rhetorician in residence," or a writing teacher who acts as a consultant and holds workshops for students that complement the existing curriculum.
- A team-taught, writing-intensive course with an occupational therapist paired with a writing specialist.
- A writer-taught, writing-intensive course with occupational therapy faculty member input in the course design,

6. Never assume that an English teacher or writing specialist knows better than you do about what your students will need to do as writers. Writing teachers are just a little more focused on writing than you are, obviously and necessarily, and they have a bit more practice with teaching this learning process. We suggest hiring someone who will help with your program's goals and not

the goals of the English department, as these goals manifest themselves in a general composition or writing course.

Teaching (With) Writing in the Field

Although we have directed the suggestions outlined to this point explicitly toward academic educators in a college or university setting, preceptors and faculty mentors may also adapt writing pedagogy during students' fieldwork experiences in clinical placements. Actually, the writing that a student undertakes in a fieldwork setting will carry with it a sense of practical realism that some school writing assignments tend to lack for students. Clinical notes, memos, letters, reports, and policy statements arise in everyday situations of therapeutic practice and, thus, in situations that occupational therapy student writers will likely encounter at some point in their future professional practice. As we implied in many of our previous suggestions, however, often even the simplest kinds of documents will be unfamiliar, and their production will be baffling at first for writers who are new to the situations in which these textual forms arise. To assist novice occupational therapists, experienced therapists may consider the following suggestions.

1. Think about and share personal experiences with learning to write in professional work. As with the other aspects of clinical practice, students enter fieldwork to learn about these practical experiences. Communicate the "nuts and bolts" as well as the thinking strategies that have been a recipe for success in this and other professional practice sites.

2. Create an archive of sample texts to read rhetorically and discuss with occupational therapy students. A preceptor may show the student a few good models of each sort of writing that is typically necessary in that particular field setting and then discuss what specifically makes each piece of writing "work well." Discuss the rhetorical development of a given text by considering such questions as the following:
   - Who is the writer?
   - How does the writer want to be perceived or understood?
   - Who is the intended reader?
   - What does the writer want the reader to do or feel?
   - What is the purpose of this text or this kind of text?
   - How can we see these elements in particular parts of the text (e.g., word choice, overall structure or format, amount of "personality" included)?
   - What does each part of the text do?

3. Review and respond constructively to drafts of students' writing in the typical forms required in this fieldwork setting. Again, remember that learning to write for a specific setting takes time, and these newcomers will be less

threatened when they have an opportunity to do some "trial runs" at new forms of writing. Likewise consider that the very newness of the clinical setting may be overwhelming in and of itself, and, when overwhelmed, a student may temporarily lose track of his or her grammatical correctness (he or she has plenty of other challenges to contend with, and spelling may be "lost in the shuffle" initially). Allowing time for rough drafts and pointing out what worked well or not so well in them will enable students to focus on what to expect in the clinical setting.

4. Engage occupational therapy students in sustained written reflection on their practice in the clinical setting. A more "narrative–processual" type of writing (e.g., a long-term, informal learning journal) may offer the students a way to record decisions and, thus, trace their development in clinical reasoning during the course of many events. A more "summative–evaluative" type of writing (e.g., a final report or self-evaluation) may enable students to draw on processual observations and to frame conclusions about their professional development. A portfolio of various kinds of writing that the student has completed, including journal entries, reports, and samples of site-specific professional writing, would allow teachers to evaluate performance in a range of activities.

Some Thoughts in Closing, Some Points of Departure

Even within one department, vastly divergent instructional world views can further complicate the already complex, multitheoried, and multi-identitied professional landscape of occupational therapy. As the occupational therapy field continues its reflections on its professional status, and on the many sorts of practice in which its members will engage in the course of their careers, certainly the practice of writing will remain a focus of attention. Writing activities within clinical situations may not substantially change, but outside of the therapeutic context, professional occupational therapy writing will be transformed, becoming more the tool of choice for occupational therapy advocacy in the many forms that this political work may assume. Certainly, occupational therapists want to communicate more effectively and powerfully for their field in the academic and professional disciplines, in public policy areas, in the health care industry, and in other local political scenes (e.g., their home universities and health care facilities). With this in mind, we leave our readers with questions to prompt further discussion rather than with conclusions about a historical process that is yet unfolding:

- What kinds of writing are occupational therapists doing now?
- How will these change as the profession changes?
- What sorts of new publications may benefit the profession and offer different avenues and audiences for occupational therapists to share their various forms of knowledge?

- What kinds of writing will better make a case for occupational therapy as a profession?
- What kinds of writing skills will make new occupational therapy graduates more employable? Effective as advocates for the profession? Autonomous in their clinical practice? Better as collaborators with other health care professionals?

We have written this article and generated these questions to attend consciously to writing as a mode of learning and of belonging to a community. Our intent is to open a conversation on the ways that faculty members may more effectively use composing for the education of new therapists. For in these students' hands (or, rather, in their pens and keyboards), many of the new worlds in occupational therapy will take shape.

Acknowledgment

Confidentiality agreements prohibit acknowledging a research site and participants by name, but we thank the institution and faculty members who participated in Detweiler's unpublished qualitative study. Their contributions have been invaluable.

This work was funded by a Junior Faculty Research Award, Office of Sponsored Projects, University of Nevada, Reno.

References

American Occupational Therapy Association/Accreditation Council for Occupational Therapy Education. (1995). *Essentials and guidelines for an accredited educational program for the occupational therapist.* Bethesda, MD: Author.

Bartholomae, D. (1985). Inventing the university. In M. Rose (Ed.), *When a writer can't write* (pp. 134–165). New York: Guilford.

Bazerman, C. (1998). *Shaping written knowledge: The genre and activity of the experimental article in science.* Madison, WI: University of Wisconsin Press.

Bazerman, C., & Paradis, J. (1991). *Textual dynamics of the professions: Historical and contemporary studies of writing in professional communities.* Madison, WI: University of Wisconsin Press.

Berkenkotter, C., & Huckin, T. (1995). *Genre knowledge in disciplinary communication: Cognition, culture, power.* New York: Erlbaum.

Berthoff, A. (1981). *The making of meaning: Metaphors, models, and maxims for writing teachers.* Montclair, NJ: Boynton/Cook.

Bizzell, P. (1982). Cognition, context, and certainty: What we need to know about writing. *Pre/Text, 3*(3), 213–243.

Brodkey, L. (1987). *Academic writing as a social practice.* Philadelphia: Temple University Press.

Elbow, P. (1973). *Writing with power: Techniques for mastering the writing process*. New York: Oxford University Press.

Elbow, P. (1981). *Writing without teachers*. New York: Oxford University Press.

Emig, J. (1981). Writing as a mode of learning. In G. Tate & E. Corbett (Eds.), *The writing teacher's sourcebook* (pp. 69–79). New York: Oxford University Press.

Herrington, A. (1985). Writing in academic settings: A study of writing in two college chemical engineering courses. *Research in the Teaching of English, 23*(2), 117–138.

Herrington, A., & Moran, C. (Eds.). (1992). *Writing, teaching, and learning in the disciplines*. New York: Modern Language Association.

Macrorie, K. (1970). *Telling writing*. New York: Hayden.

Pierce, D., & Peyton, C. (1999). A historical cross-disciplinary perspective on the professional doctorate in occupational therapy. *American Journal of Occupational Therapy, 53*, 64–72.

Prior, P. (1991). Contextualizing writing and response in a graduate seminar. *Written Communication, 8*(3), 267–310.

Prior, P. (1995). Tracing authoritative and internally persuasive discourses: A case study of response, revision, and disciplinary enculturation. *Research in the Teaching of English, 29*(3), 288–325.

Quiroga, V. (1995). *Occupational therapy: The first 30 years, 1900–1930*. Bethesda, MD: American Occupational Therapy Association.

PROBLEM-BASED LEARNING
AND CLINICAL REASONING

A Review of the Problem-Based Learning Literature in Occupational Therapy

Lori Caterina
Perri Stern

Lori Caterina, MOT, is Traumatic Brain and Spinal Cord Injury State Program Coordinator, University Affiliated Center for Developmental Disabilities, Robert C. Byrd Health Sciences Center, West Virginia University, Morgantown, West Virginia.

Perri Stern, EdD, OTR, is Assistant Department Chair, Department of Occupational Therapy, Rangos School of Health Sciences at Duquesne University, Pittsburgh, Pennsylvania.

The desire to "bridge the gap" between theory and practice in occupational therapy has led to the implementation of problem-based learning (PBL) in many occupational therapy curricula. To date, no systematic review of the literature has determined the current state of PBL in occupational therapy education. The purpose of the following review was to determine how the occupational therapy literature has described PBL and where future research is necessary. Descriptions of PBL are comprehensive, whereas outcomes are inconclusive and are merely a reflection of the medical literature. Educators should pursue research directed toward providing evidence to validate this educational practice.

The desire to "bridge the gap" between theory and practice in allied health has led to the implementation of problem-based learning (PBL) in many occupational therapy curricula (Jacobs, 1997a; Sadlo, Piper, & Agnew, 1994; Steward, 1996). Descriptions and accounts of PBL appeared in the occupational therapy literature as early as 1983 (Cooper, 1983). The literature has included discussion regarding the methods to educate students to identify and solve problems in occupational therapy as far back as 1969 (Line, 1969). However, to date, no systematic review of the literature has determined the current state of PBL in occupational therapy education.

The purpose of this study was to determine what knowledge currently exists in occupational therapy regarding PBL. A review and analysis of the existing literature from 1969 to the present determined how the occupational therapy literature has articulated PBL during the past 30 years. This article provides comprehensive information regarding the "state of the art" of an educational strategy that has received increasing attention, especially in recent years. This article also provides occupational therapy educators with a critical summary of what we know about PBL and direction and focus for further research.

The following research questions guided this study:

- What areas of emphasis exist within the occupational therapy literature related to PBL?
- How thoroughly has the literature discussed these areas?
- What issues has the literature not addressed?

PBL

PBL emerged in medical education in 1963, largely on the basis of the work of H. S. Barrows. Barrows observed that medical students were capable of conducting a patient history and of carrying out a routine medical examination; however, in general, students were unable to *apply* knowledge across diverse situations

(Barrows & Tamblyn as cited by Savin-Baden, 1997a). The demand for greater accountability within education and potential employers' expectations for graduates to possess problem-solving skills on entering the job market likewise influenced the advent of PBL in medical education (Savin-Baden, 1997a).

PBL does not refer to one specific educational method (Barrows, 1986). PBL refers to a group of teaching and learning methods and reflects a set of beliefs about teaching and learning processes. PBL aims to enhance students' functional knowledge and to promote self-directed skills for inquiry and internal motivation for learning. In addition, PBL aims to increase students' abilities to evaluate their learning needs, strengths, and limitations (Walton & Matthews, 1989). According to Barrows (1986), authentic PBL should meet four specific objectives in health care education:

1. Structuring knowledge for use in clinical contexts
2. Developing clinical reasoning skills
3. Increasing self-directed learning
4. Fostering motivation for learning

Literature related to PBL in medical education is comprehensive. Numerous articles and books have provided definitions of PBL, described the educational rationale that supports PBL, discussed implementation issues, and reported on various outcomes (Albanese & Mitchell, 1993).

Methods

We conducted a literature search through MEDLINE, CINAHL, and ERIC for the years 1966 to 1998. Key words used to search each database included *problem-based learning*, *self-directed learning*, and *case-based learning*, each in conjunction with occupational therapy. Current Contents obtained any recent publications that were not in the databases. We reviewed each article and used only those that specifically referred to PBL as Barrows (1986) defined it.

We first analyzed articles to determine the areas of content throughout the PBL literature in occupational therapy. After we identified these content areas, we examined each article more closely to determine how thoroughly each area was discussed. We drew parallels among the articles. Finally, we analyzed the data to determine which content areas the literature has not discussed and where future research is necessary.

We located 36 articles of which 28 met Barrows' (1986) criteria and were included in this study. These 28 articles ultimately yielded six major categories:

1. Issues in occupational therapy education
2. Curriculum design
3. Implementation strategies

4. Student perceptions
   5. Faculty development
   6. Outcomes

Table 1 summarizes which articles addressed each of these categories.

Issues in Occupational Therapy Education

Five articles described the influential factors that have instigated changes within occupational therapy education (Jacobs, 1997a; Royeen, 1995; Sadlo et al., 1994; Savin-Baden, 1997a; Watson & West, 1996). Each of these authors identified PBL as a response to changes in health care.

Jacobs (1997a) and Savin-Baden (1997a) attributed changes in education to various issues, including economic constraints, changing governmental policies, increased emphasis on quality assurance, accountability of the clinician, increased employer expectations for graduates, and rapidly increasing technology. However, the philosophies and practices that graduates are expected to develop and relay to the next generation do not always match the content of undergraduate education (Savin-Baden, 1997a). Royeen (1995) discussed several issues related to occupational therapy education, including the following:

- The need for occupational therapists to apply principles, theories, and approaches to the dynamic functional problems that persons with disabilities encounter
- The need to work within the context of today's constantly changing society
- The need to recognize occupational therapy's potential to serve persons of all backgrounds with and without disabilities

Traditionally, aside from fieldwork education, occupational therapy education has focused primarily on lecture and involves separate academic subjects. Course content has focused on the patient, is often disease oriented, and involves the medical model (Jacobs, 1997a; Sadlo et al., 1994; Watson & West, 1996). Clinical skills and abilities usually develop during fieldwork after students gain knowledge through lectures and textbooks. Students are expected to learn vast amounts of information in an attempt to keep up with the rapidly increasing amount of information that is available. Many believe that this format is ineffective because "it emphasizes the need to know what is known today, and not how we should learn for what will be known tomorrow" (Sadlo et al., 1994, p. 49).

Several authors have critiqued traditional occupational therapy education (Jacobs, 1997a; Sadlo et al., 1994; Savin-Baden, 1997a). According to these authors, within many traditional educational formats, a lack of meaningfulness and relevance exists for students (according to clinicians), and this format does not promote many of the desired attributes of occupational therapy graduates.

Table 1
Articles Addressing Major Categories in Occupational Therapy PBL Literature

Category	Citations
Issues in occupational therapy education	Jacobs, 1997a; Royeen, 1995; Sadlo, Piper, & Agnew, 1994; Savin-Baden, 1997a; Watson & West, 1996
Curriculum design	Bruhn, 1992; Busuttil, 1996; Jacobs, 1997a; Royeen, 1995; Royeen & Salvatori, 1997; Saarinen & Salvatori, 1994; Sadlo, 1994; Sadlo et al., 1994; Watson & West, 1996; Westmorland, Salvatori, Tremblay, Jung, & Martin, 1996
Implementation strategies	Cooper, 1983; Hay, 1995, 1997a, 1997b; Jacobs, 1997a, 1997b; Royeen, 1995; Royeen & Salvatori, 1997; Saarinen & Salvatori, 1994; Sadlo, 1994; Sadlo et al., 1994; Stern, 1997; Urbina, Hess, Andrews, Hammond, & Clark, 1997; VanLeit, 1995; Watson & West, 1996; Westmorland et al., 1996
Student perceptions	Jacobs, 1997b; Saarinen & Salvatori, 1994; Sadlo, 1994; Savin-Baden, 1997b, 1998; Stern, 1997; Westmorland et al., 1996; Williams, Saarinen-Rahikka, & Norman, 1995
Faculty development	Brandon & Majumdar, 1997; Hay, 1996, 1997a, 1997b; Royeen & Salvatori, 1997; Sadlo et al., 1994; Stern, 1998; Watson & West, 1996
Outcomes	Bruhn, 1997; Hay, 1995; Royeen & Salvatori, 1997; Saarinen & Salvatori, 1994; Sadlo et al., 1994; Watson & West, 1996; Williams et al., 1995

Such attributes include the ability to integrate theoretical knowledge with clinical skills and analytical thinking, problem-solving, and imaginative skills. Watson and West (1996) cited Barrows (1985), who argued that

> the use of lectures in an educational curriculum is inversely related to attaining self-directed skills, structuring knowledge for the use in clinical contexts, developing effective clinical reasoning processes, and increasing student motivation for learning. (p. 83)

Occupational therapy education must emphasize the preparation of students for many years of practice and lifelong learning (Royeen, 1995; Sadlo et al., 1994). Royeen (1995) believed that an educational foundation in clinical reasoning and critical reflection is essential. She cited Ross (1989), who developed a synopsis of the stages of critical reflection and clinical reasoning. Royeen (1995) also cited Roth (1989), who described the critical reflection process as involving certain attitudes and abilities, including introspection, open-mindedness, accepting responsibility, viewing problems from different perspectives, and using data to support or validate a decision. What we must determine is how to educate occupational therapists in these competencies.

Watson and West (1996) believed that successful professionals in the new health care environment need to identify and resolve problems to improve quality and cost outcomes, to work effectively in teams to support comprehensive service delivery, to manage complex and expanding information and technology, and to participate actively in a diverse workforce. Watson and West stated that education that aims to address the requirements of this environment would focus on group-centered learning, inquiry, research, and multimedia resource access. Education should also focus on the process of learning, active learning, an environment in which learners direct and evaluate themselves, and the promotion of lifelong learning.

Four articles discussed the principles of PBL and their relationship to the current goals of occupational therapy education (Jacobs, 1997a; Sadlo et al., 1994; Savin-Baden, 1997a; Stern, 1997). According to these authors, PBL uses adult learning principles, integrates theory and practice, and makes course content meaningful to students. In addition, through PBL, students develop skills for lifelong, self-directed learning that enhance their clinical reasoning skills and capacities for synthesizing course content across the curriculum. PBL likewise enhances students' commitment to teamwork and professional development and emphasizes integrating ideas and principles to promote the student's ability to keep pace with new information in health care.

Mohawk College in Hamilton, Ontario, was one of the first schools to base its occupational therapy program on a PBL format. On the basis of the school's educational goals, its philosophy of occupational therapy, and the health needs of Canadians, the Mohawk curriculum focused on developing clinicians with problem-solving skills (Jacobs, 1997a; Westmorland, Salvatori, Tremblay, Jung, & Martin, 1996). Three articles discussed the parallel between educational program goals and the principles of PBL regarding the development of several other occupational therapy programs (Royeen & Salvatori, 1997; Sadlo et al., 1994; Stern, 1997).

VanLeit (1995) discussed the connection between clinical reasoning and PBL. She cited Fleming (1991), who described the procedural, interactive, and conditional clinical reasoning tracks that therapists use. VanLeit discussed the potential for education to address clinical reasoning through PBL by designing specific cases to illustrate each clinical reasoning tract.

Curriculum Design

The literature has described various occupational therapy programs with a PBL format. Most of these programs are 2 to 3 years in length and result in either a baccalaureate degree or a master's degree. These programs include McMaster University in Hamilton, Ontario (Royeen & Salvatori, 1997; Saarinen & Salvatori, 1994; Watson & West, 1996; Westmorland et al., 1996); Shenandoah University in Winchester, Virginia (Royeen, 1995; Royeen & Salvatori, 1997); the University of Newcastle in Callaghan, New South Wales, Australia (Bruhn, 1992; Jacobs, 1997a; Watson & West, 1996); the West London Institute, Brunel University College in London (Sadlo, 1994; Sadlo et al., 1994); the Occupational Therapy School in Malta (Busuttil, 1996); and the University of New Mexico in Albuquerque (Watson & West, 1996). Watson and West (1996) provided a comprehensive comparison of programs at five universities that offer a PBL occupational therapy program. Royeen and Salvatori (1997) provided a comparison between the PBL programs at Shenandoah University and McMaster University. Royeen (1995) described the logistical steps that Shenandoah University undertook in the development of a PBL curriculum for its occupational therapy program.

Included in each article is a discussion of how course content is organized within the program. Study may revolve around PBL units, life span thematic blocks, thematic units, learning units, or content blocks. Although the curriculum structure varies somewhat from one program to the next, each PBL unit is designed to meet specific learning objectives. Royeen (1995) provided four dimensions of learning objectives that each PBL unit addresses:

1. Knowledge and understanding
2. Interpersonal attributes and skills
3. Clinical skills
4. Clinical reasoning

Jacobs (1997a) developed a schematic approach to encourage the integration of PBL in occupational therapy curricula. Her approach essentially has two levels. The first level shows how knowledge and skills acquired through subject bases, such as bioscience, research, and occupation and activity, are integrated into the philosophy, theories, concepts, and beliefs of the profession of occupational therapy. This process of integration defines the progress of the field and the development of occupational therapy practitioners.

The second level provides an approach to the problems used for learning. Here, a specific intervention issue is surrounded by a range of fundamental occupational therapy concepts and subject streams among which the student must integrate related knowledge and skills to meet course objectives and to develop potential solutions to the problem. This system focuses on the holistic approach that is implicit in PBL. The development of courses around this schema enables students to accumulate knowledge, to analyze problems critically, and to develop practical skills simultaneously.

Richardson, Cooper, Swanson, and Ward (1995), Saarinen and Salvatori (1994), Sadlo (1994), and Watson and West (1996) each emphasized the importance of interdisciplinary learning. Several curricula provide opportunities for occupational therapy, physical therapy, and nursing students to work and learn together in a PBL format. The experience of working with other disciplines prepares students for a clinical environment in which success relies heavily on one's ability to communicate and collaborate with other health care professionals.

Fieldwork may occur after learning units, within thematic blocks, or across the curriculum (Watson & West, 1996). Four articles (Jacobs, 1997a; Saarinen & Salvatori, 1994; Watson & West, 1996; Westmorland et al., 1996) specifically discussed how the systematic timing of fieldwork can allow the student to integrate immediately knowledge and skills acquired in a clinical setting. In fieldwork, "the focus of student learning shifts from paper scenarios to actual clients" (Saarinen & Salvatori, 1994, p. 85).

Several authors described the format and process of a PBL course (Jacobs, 1997a; Royeen, 1995; Saarinen & Salvatori, 1994; Sadlo, 1994; Sadlo et al., 1994; Stern, 1997; VanLeit, 1995; Watson & West, 1996). Information included tutorial group size and format, qualifications for group facilitators, frequency of meetings, and course objectives. Group size ranged from 6 to 15 students, with 1 faculty member or therapist serving as a group facilitator. Groups typically meet for 2 to 6 hr a week. Five articles included information on tutorial formats. Stern (1997) provided a comprehensive summary of the process.

Implementation Strategies

Seven articles specifically discussed the role of the tutor in the PBL curriculum (Hay, 1997a, 1997b; Royeen & Salvatori, 1997; Saarinen & Salvatori, 1994; Sadlo, 1994; Sadlo et al., 1994; Stern, 1997). Tutors are most often faculty members or occupational therapists from the community. According to Sadlo et al. (1994), "The tutor's role is to guide and encourage, to challenge and question, and to facilitate the development of concepts, not to dispense information or to direct the group's progress too much" (p. 51). Tutors create an atmosphere of shared learning and avoid negative judgment that can cause anxiety in the student and may interfere with the learning process (Sadlo, 1994). Tutors probe to establish an appropriate depth of knowledge, to monitor student dynamics, and to evaluate student performance (Saarinen & Salvatori, 1994). Tutors provide feedback to the group and to the individual regarding problem-solving, teamwork, independent thinking, clinical reasoning, and professional skills (Hay, 1997a, 1997b; Saarinen & Salvatori, 1994; Stern, 1997).

Information related to cases included sources, format, content, and guidelines for case construction. Five articles discussed potential sources for PBL cases (Jacobs, 1997a; Sadlo, 1994; Sadlo et al., 1994; Stern, 1997; Urbina, Hess, Andrews, Hammond, & Clark, 1997). Faculty members, occupational therapists in the community, and students have developed cases. For example, at Virginia Commonwealth University in Richmond, Virginia, occupational therapists representing different specialty and practice areas as well as social workers were consulted to identify appropriate cases in their practices (Stern, 1997).

Articles have also described specific options for formatting cases (Cooper, 1983; Sadlo et al., 1994; VanLeit, 1995; Westmorland et al., 1996). PBL cases may be presented on paper or by using videotape with simulated clients or real clients. At McMaster University, cases have been presented as clinical problems packaged like a deck of cards (P-4 decks) (Cooper, 1983; Westmorland et al., 1996).

Case content may include signs and symptoms of a disease, one or two main issues involving a client, a synopsis of the overall situation, sample occupational therapy evaluation and treatment plans, information from the medical chart, a description of functional limitations, and helpful resources for information (Royeen, 1995; Sadlo, 1994; Stern, 1997; Watson & West, 1996; Urbina et al., 1997).

Guidelines for writing cases (Jacobs, 1997a; Royeen, 1995; Sadlo et al., 1994; Urbina et al., 1997; Watson & West, 1996) have suggested incorporating perspectives from different disciplines and addressing a continuum of care encompassing the client, the family members, the community, and public policy (Urbina et al., 1997). Cases should stimulate clinical reasoning and require the student to understand scientific information related to the case and to apply occupational therapy theoretical models or frames of reference (Royeen, 1995; Watson & West, 1996). Cases must be constructed in such a way as to ensure that students can generalize concepts that they learn to various clients (Jacobs, 1997a). According to Watson and West (1996),

> Problems portrayed are realistic, provide a trigger for learning, create a relevant context for knowledge and skill development, prepare students intellectually and emotionally for the clinical situations they will encounter, and require learners to practice all of the cognitive steps and professional behaviors required of reflective practitioners. (p. 84)

Ten articles discussed the various methods to evaluate student performance (Hay, 1995; Jacobs, 1997b; Royeen, 1995; Royeen & Salvatori, 1997; Saarinen & Salvatori, 1994; Sadlo, 1994; Sadlo et al., 1994; Stern, 1997; Watson & West, 1996; Westmorland et al., 1996). Students are evaluated via traditional means, such as testing and written assignments (Royeen & Salvatori, 1997; Sadlo, 1994; Stern, 1997; Watson & West, 1996); innovative tutor, peer, and self-evaluations; and a practical examination.

Jacobs (1997b) described the evaluation methods at the University of Newcastle. She stated that evaluation should follow PBL principles and should not include traditional methods of examination: "The assessment developed in Newcastle enables students to practice the same skills that they will be required to perform in the real world" (p. 175).

Common in the literature is discussion of the use of peer, faculty member, and self-evaluations of student performance in the group setting (Royeen, 1995; Royeen & Salvatori, 1997; Saarinen & Salvatori, 1994; Sadlo, 1994; Sadlo et al., 1994; Watson & West, 1996). Virginia Commonwealth University uses a 15-item self-, peer, and faculty rating form to address students' use of professional language and behaviors; quality of questions; sensitivity to complex ethical, cultural, or clinical issues; and factual knowledge related to the case at hand (Stern, 1997). Students also answer two open-ended questions to elicit individual learning goals:

> The rationale for this multi-perspective evaluation system was for students to have the opportunity to give and receive feedback in a way that simulated some of the feedback they would be expected to give and receive in a professional or clinical setting. (Stern, 1997, p. 592)

Five articles described the use of the Triple Jump exercise as a method of evaluation (Jacobs, 1997b; Sadlo et al., 1994; Stern, 1997; Watson & West, 1996; Westmorland et al., 1996). The Triple Jump is typically a three-part examination to evaluate students' independent thinking and clinical reasoning skills (Sadlo et al., 1994; Stern, 1997; Westmorland et al., 1996). During this examination, instructors evaluate students on their ability to demonstrate competence with the PBL process independently. Advocates of the Triple Jump note the importance of this individual aspect of PBL.

The issue of grading in a PBL curriculum raises some debate among PBL proponents. In a pure PBL approach, students often receive no grades (Royeen, 1995). However, several factors make the use of grades necessary. First, grades are important for admission to further graduate study (Royeen & Salvatori, 1997; Saarinen & Salvatori, 1994). Second, programs use grades because of institutional requirements (Royeen & Salvatori, 1997). Grades can provide useful feedback for students by assisting them to identify personal strengths and weaknesses. Some programs have managed to negotiate this issue successfully. For example, at Shenandoah University, students receive traditional grades for knowledge and understanding (Royeen, 1995; Watson & West, 1996). All other content block objectives are evaluated on a pass or fail basis. Students must receive a passing mark in the areas of interpersonal attributes, clinical skills, and clinical reasoning before they are eligible to receive letter grades for knowledge and understanding.

Student Perceptions

The literature on student perceptions and experiences with PBL has included results from course evaluations and student interviews (Jacobs, 1997b; Saarinen & Salvatori, 1994; Sadlo, 1994; Savin-Baden, 1997b, 1998; Stern, 1997; Westmorland et al., 1996; Williams, Saarinen-Rahikka, & Norman, 1995).

Discussion has focused on students' perceptions of the strengths and weaknesses of PBL. Stern (1997) completed a study at Virginia Commonwealth University in which students were interviewed at the end of a 7-week PBL course and 6 weeks after the course during Level II fieldwork. During these interviews, students reflected on their perceptions of the course after they made the transition from the classroom to a clinical setting. Stern's findings indicated that students believed that PBL enhanced their professional behavior, prepared them for clinical fieldwork, enhanced their clinical reasoning skills, contributed to their self-confidence during fieldwork, and fostered their pursuit of self-directed learning.

At McMaster University, students complete an exit survey. They have the opportunity to reflect on the perceived strengths and weaknesses of the program. The university conducts graduate tracking to receive additional feedback from former students and current employers (Saarinen & Salvatori, 1994; Westmorland et al., 1996).

Sadlo (1994), Westmorland et al. (1996), and Saarinen and Salvatori (1994) discussed the perceived strengths of PBL curricula according to students. Strengths included self-directed learning, small group learning, the variety of clinical practice settings encountered, the use of clinicians for teaching, integration of content in the tutorials with clinical skills, labs, and overall relevance of learning. Overall, students found PBL to be motivating and were confident in their clinical reasoning skills. Ninety-one percent of the students in a study that Sadlo (1994) conducted had a positive view of PBL. Students noted some weaknesses, including limited application of basic sciences (e.g., physics, anatomy), a heavy course load, and limited opportunities for skill development.

Savin-Baden (1997b, 1998) extensively discussed a study that examined the expectations and experiences of students using PBL. The author described how students made sense of PBL's purposes, processes, and outcomes. Savin-Baden (1998) identified learning paradoxes that were apparent in PBL: "PBL can be a catalyst to different forms of disjunction for different students at different times and in diverse programs in professional education which use PBL as a focus for learning" (p. 14).

Faculty Development

A limited amount of information exists in the literature regarding training and development activities for PBL faculty members. Stern (1998) described a four-session faculty development workshop project for academic and fieldwork educators associated with the Occupational Therapy Department at Duquesne University in Pittsburgh, Pennsylvania.

The goals for this workshop were to provide academic and fieldwork educators with an in-depth orientation to PBL and to recruit potential tutors for a planned PBL segment of an existing course. Participants received an orientation to PBL principles and details about specific components of a PBL course and became immersed in the PBL group process. By experiencing the PBL process, the group members were able to explore potential difficulties that may arise in a tutorial session and to identify options for implementing aspects of PBL into daily practice.

Three articles by Hay (1996, 1997a, 1997b) discussed tutor evaluation in PBL. The author described a 19-item instrument with which students evaluated their PBL tutor. The evaluation contained specific performance aspects and provided a global rating for the tutor. According to Hay (1997a), "Tutor evaluations commonly provide both formative and summative feedback. Formative feedback provides tutors with an opportunity to modify their actions during the course to better meet the students' needs" (p. 141).

Throughout the PBL literature in occupational therapy, the need for PBL tutors with content expertise has stirred debate (Brandon & Majumdar, 1997; Royeen & Salvatori, 1997; Sadlo et al., 1994; Watson & West, 1996). According to Sadlo et al. (1994),

> Tutors do not need to be experienced in the field being studied, because non-experts are able to focus more on the group process and less on directing the content. However, students may be most satisfied with expert tutors who can remain non-directive. (p. 51)

Brandon and Majumdar (1997) stated that although expert tutors may be able to ask more probing questions, they may likewise provide knowledge to students, which may ultimately affect the PBL process.

Outcomes

Seven articles presented outcomes of PBL (Bruhn, 1997; Hay, 1995; Royeen & Salvatori, 1997; Saarinen & Salvatori, 1994; Sadlo et al., 1994; Watson & West, 1996; Williams et al., 1995). However, view these data with caution because most of the outcomes in the occupational therapy literature result from research in medical education. We must be careful about applying these results to occupational therapy education.

Limited evidence exists to support PBL (Saarinen & Salvatori, 1994), but PBL may increase knowledge retention, enhance students' abilities to transfer concepts to new problems, and promote students' abilities to integrate basic sciences into clinical practice (Saarinen & Salvatori, 1994; Sadlo et al., 1994). PBL graduates tend to receive higher ratings from their clinical supervisors, appear more motivated, and develop desired deep-learning approaches (Sadlo et al., 1994).

According to Sadlo et al. (1994), the medical literature has suggested that clinical reasoning develops more quickly during work with problems. Evidence suggests that reasoning and problem-solving abilities are more efficient in PBL students; however, whether problem solving is a skill that can be taught is not known (Royeen & Salvatori, 1997; Sadlo et al., 1994). PBL does seem to increase self-directed behaviors, enhance student interest in subject matter, and promote the development of lifelong learning skills (Royeen & Salvatori, 1997; Saarinen & Salvatori, 1994; Watson & West, 1996).

> We believe that PBL provides a realistic and humanistic context for learning, improves lifelong learning skills, and parallels occupational therapy's tradition of meaningful engagement, holistic analysis, and the promotion of independent performance. (Watson & West, 1996, p. 91)

Two studies discussed outcomes related to occupational therapy PBL programs (Hay, 1995; Williams et al., 1995). Hay (1995) completed a study that compared occupational therapy students' self-evaluations of their performances with the evaluations they received from their tutors in a PBL course. The study investigated whether repeated opportunities for students to evaluate their performance formally during tutorials assisted the development of self-evaluation skills. However, the results of the study indicated that students and faculty members became more adept at negotiating ratings versus increasing agreement on tutorial performance.

Williams et al. (1995) researched the amount of time that PBL students spent on educational activities and sought to determine whether the amount of time increased or decreased as students progressed through the program. This study showed a general decrease in time spent in educational activities, and the authors hypothesized that this reflected familiarity with course expectations and increased efficiency in using learning resources.

Where Do We Go From Here?

Clearly, within occupational therapy, PBL research must focus on outcomes. Since 1994, numerous authors have articulated this urgent need (Bruhn, 1997; Royeen & Salvatori, 1997; Sadlo, 1994; Sadlo et al., 1994). According to Sadlo et al. (1994),

> Lack of comprehensive evaluative studies, apprehensions of cost and disruption, lack of experience with the process, and the disbelief that students will acquire

knowledge as effectively as in 'taught' courses remain obstacles to a wider adoption. (p. 54)

To determine whether PBL is effective, we must develop valid methods of measuring knowledge and clinical outcomes (Bruhn, 1997). The existing studies, which only reflect the medical literature, are inconclusive because of methodological problems that are inherent when comparing PBL curricula and traditional curricula (Solomon, 1994). Evaluation methods should adapt to the profession of occupational therapy and its philosophical underpinnings. Neither applying medically based outcome data or outcome measures to a field that is moving away from the medical model nor comparing the learning methods of medical students with those of occupational therapy students seems reasonable.

One main concern is that students in a PBL curriculum do not perform as well in the basic sciences and lack confidence in these subjects (Sadlo et al., 1994). According to Royeen and Salvatori (1997), initial learning may be less than with traditional instruction, but knowledge retention increases. Sadlo et al. (1994) stated, "The role of 'basic' knowledge in clinical performance is still not fully understood by educators, and the correct tutorial methods for reinforcing knowledge are not always practiced" (p. 52). Clearly, research is necessary in these areas.

Another area for research involves the cost-effectiveness of PBL efforts (Brandon & Majumdar, 1997; Sadlo, 1994; Sadlo et al., 1994; Watson & West, 1996). Although whether PBL courses are more expensive than traditional courses is not known, an increased demand for resources is evident in PBL, such as library facilities to support self-directed learning and physical space for small group sessions. Increased costs are most likely incurred with larger class sizes (greater than 100 students) because of the number of faculty members necessary to facilitate small groups. Some authors suggested that the time commitment of faculty members is no greater in a PBL curriculum (Brandon & Majumdar, 1997; Watson & West, 1996). However, Sadlo (1994) stated that

the course has proved no more expensive to run than subject-based curriculum, although staff commitment needs to be high in order to develop the problems, and to ensure the success of a process which is new and evolving. (p. 83)

Studies should determine whether PBL is a cost-effective method of education in terms of financial issues and personnel.

Given PBL's emphasis on independent, self-directed, lifelong learning, studies to evaluate the development of students' research strategies would be beneficial in evaluating the development of these skills.

Finally, longitudinal studies are necessary to document PBL students' abilities to structure knowledge in clinical contexts and to develop effective clinical reasoning skills. Research should focus on comparing students from a PBL curriculum with students from a traditional curriculum at graduation and 5 to

10 years later, after they have had the opportunity to implement lifelong, self-directed learning skills.

Conclusions

PBL has received increasing and consistent attention in occupational therapy education. The results of this literature review reveal a wealth of information about program design, case format, educational rationale, and implementation strategies. However, a dearth of information exists regarding specific PBL outcomes. Occupational therapy educators should be encouraged by the interest in developing innovative educational methods that promote the essential qualities of tomorrow's occupational therapists. However, just as clinicians must provide research evidence that validates their clinical practice, educators must respond to this same call and pursue research directed toward providing such evidence for this educational practice.

References

Albanese, M. A., & Mitchell, S. (1993). Problem-based learning: A review of the literature on its outcomes and implementation issues. *Academic Medicine, 68*(1), 52–81.

Barrows, H. S. (1986). A taxonomy of problem-based learning methods. *Medical Education, 20*, 481–486.

Brandon, J. E., & Majumdar, B. (1997). An introduction and evaluation of problem-based learning in health professions education. *Family and Community Health, 20*(1), 1–15.

Bruhn, J. G. (1992). Problem-based learning: An approach toward reforming allied health education. *Journal of Allied Health, 21*(3), 161–173.

Bruhn, J. G. (1997). Outcomes of problem-based learning in health care professional education: A critique. *Family and Community Health, 20*(1), 66–74.

Busuttil, J. (1996). A problem-based learning occupational therapy course: The second year. *British Journal of Occupational Therapy, 59*, 8–10.

Cooper, B. A. (1983). The P-4 deck (portable patient problem pack): Educational tool of the future? *Canadian Journal of Occupational Therapy, 50*, 21–24.

Hay, J. A. (1995). Investigating the development of self-evaluation skills in a problem-based tutorial course. *Academic Medicine, 70*, 733–735.

Hay, J. A. (1996). An examination of a tutor evaluation form for problem-based learning curricula in physical therapy and occupational therapy education. *Journal of Physical Therapy Education, 10*(1), 22–25.

Hay, J. A. (1997a). Brief or New—An investigation of a tutor evaluation scale for formative purposes in a problem-based learning curriculum. *American Journal of Occupational Therapy, 51*, 140–143.

Hay, J. A. (1997b). Test–retest reliability of a tutor evaluation form used in a problem-based curriculum. *Canadian Journal of Occupational Therapy, 64*, 203–206.

Jacobs, T. (1997a). Developing integrated education programmes for occupational therapy: The problem of subject streams in a problem-based course. *British Journal of Occupational Therapy, 60*, 134–138.

Jacobs, T. (1997b). Integrating assessment in problem-focused curricula. *British Journal of Occupational Therapy, 60*, 174–178.

Line, J. (1969). Case method as a scientific form of clinical thinking. *American Journal of Occupational Therapy, 23*, 308–313.

Richardson, J. A., Cooper, B., Swanson, L., & Ward, M. (1995). Interprofessional education in gerontology: A problem-based model. *Geronotology and Geriatrics Education, 16*, 37–51.

Royeen, C. B. (1995). A problem-based learning curriculum for occupational therapy education. *American Journal of Occupational Therapy, 49*, 338–346.

Royeen, C. B., & Salvatori, P. (1997). Comparison of problem-based learning curricula in two occupational therapy programmes. *Canadian Journal of Occupational Therapy, 64*, 197–202.

Saarinen, H., & Salvatori, P. (1994). Educating occupational and physiotherapists for the year 2000: What, no anatomy course? *Physiotherapy Canada, 46*, 81–86.

Sadlo, G. (1994). Problem-based learning in the development of an occupational therapy curriculum: Part 2: The BSc at the London School of Occupational Therapy. *British Journal of Occupational Therapy, 57*, 79–84.

Sadlo, G., Piper, D. W., & Agnew, P. (1994). Problem-based learning in the development of an occupational therapy curriculum: Part 1: The process of problem-based learning. *British Journal of Occupational Therapy, 57*, 49–54.

Savin-Baden, M. (1997a). Problem-based learning: Part 1: An innovation whose time has come? *British Journal of Occupational Therapy, 60*, 447–450.

Savin-Baden, M. (1997b). Problem-based learning: Part 2: Understanding learner stances. *British Journal of Occupational Therapy, 60*, 531–536.

Savin-Baden, M. (1998). Problem-based learning: Part 3: Making sense of and managing disjunction. *British Journal of Occupational Therapy, 61*, 13–16.

Solomon, P. (1994). Problem-based learning: A direction for physical therapy education? *Physiotherapy Theory and Practice, 10*, 45–52.

Stern, P. (1997). Student perceptions of a problem-based learning course. *American Journal of Occupational Therapy, 51*, 589–596.

Stern, P. (1998). Brief or New—Skills for teaching: A problem-based learning faculty development workshop. *American Journal of Occupational Therapy, 52*, 230–233.

Steward, B. (1996). The theory/practice divide: Bridging the gap in occupational therapy. *British Journal of Occupational Therapy, 59*, 264–268.

Urbina, C., Hess, D., Andrews, R., Hammond, R., & Clark, H. (1997). Problem-based learning in an interdisciplinary setting. *Family and Community Health, 20*(1), 16–28.

VanLeit, B. (1995). Using the case method to develop clinical reasoning skills in problem-based learning. *American Journal of Occupational Therapy, 49*, 349–353.

Walton, H. J., & Matthews, M. B. (1989). Essentials of problem-based learning. *Medical Education, 23,* 542–558.

Watson, D. E., & West, D. J. (1996). Using problem-based learning to improve educational outcomes. *Occupational Therapy International, 3*(2), 81–93.

Westmorland, M., Salvatori, P., Tremblay, M., Jung, B., & Martin, A. (1996). The once and future programme: Educational innovation in occupational therapy. *Canadian Journal of Occupational Therapy, 63*, 44–54.

Williams, R., Saarinen-Rahikka, H., & Norman, G. R. (1995). Self-directed learning in problem-based health sciences education. *Academic Medicine, 70*(2), 161–163.

PROBLEM-BASED LEARNING AND CLINICAL REASONING

Essentials for Successful Integration of Problem-Based Learning in Occupational Therapy Curricula

Betsy VanLeit
Terry K. Crowe
Robert Waterman

Betsy VanLeit, PhD, OTR/L, was Lecturer II, Department of Orthopaedics, Occupational Therapy Program, Terry K. Crowe, PhD, OTR/L, FAOTA, is Associate Professor and Director, Occupational Therapy Program, and Robert Waterman, PhD, is Professor Emeritus, Department of Anatomy, School of Medicine, University of New Mexico, Albuquerque, New Mexico.

Occupational therapy educators are turning to problem-based learning (PBL) to facilitate student development of clinical reasoning skills, communication competencies, and lifelong learning. The University of New Mexico Occupational Therapy Program has found that successful PBL implementation requires attention to the following considerations or essentials: the need for small student groups, clear faculty roles and unified faculty attitudes, supported facilitators, independent student learning time, available learning resources, well-written and current cases, thoughtful case and curriculum development, student evaluation that is congruent with PBL methods, and integration of PBL outcomes into program evaluation. This article describes these essentials in detail and discusses issues related to implementation of PBL.

Problem-Based Learning and Occupational Therapy

The problem-based learning (PBL) philosophy is congruent with occupational therapy's belief that persons learn best through engagement in meaningful occupation (Watson & West, 1996). PBL requires that students actively participate in problem-solving and decision-making activities similar to those that occupational therapy practitioners perform. In addition, students in PBL gain experience in working as part of a team, and they have many opportunities to practice communication and feedback skills. Finally, occupational therapy's emphasis on the importance of the dynamic interaction of occupation, environment, and person parallels the PBL integrated learning approach through cases. Students naturally begin to consider client needs in the context of cases that simulate realistic client scenarios.

To become competent clinicians, occupational therapy students must develop clinical reasoning skills, effective communication abilities, and a penchant for lifelong learning. Research has identified PBL as an educational method that may facilitate all of these competencies (Shin, Haynes, & Johnston, 1993; Stern, 1997). Peterson (1998) discussed three important criteria that enable PBL to promote learning:

1. An environment in which students are immersed in a practical learning process
2. Opportunities for students to receive guidance, feedback, and support from their peers and instructors
3. Learning scenarios that involve solving "real" problems

He stressed that the success of PBL depends on the ability of students to work together to identify and analyze problems and generate solutions. Barrows (1994) believed that PBL is concerned with not only what students learn, but also how they learn in the light of their future professional tasks and responsibilities.

The notion that students need a certain amount of knowledge before they can learn to be problem solvers is a misunderstanding of the process. In fact, students already have considerable knowledge that they may only need to structure and activate (Margetson, 1996). PBL may enhance the transfer of concepts to new cases and the integration of basic science concepts into clinical scenarios (Norman & Schmidt, 1992). Any group can enjoy working together as long as the case does not require too much technical or specialized knowledge to which the students have never been exposed in any capacity. Remember that PBL draws on the life experiences of all of the participants. Even young students may have knowledge of health problems through family, work, or volunteer experiences.

Enjoyment and growth are most apt to occur through PBL if students have opportunities to practice across the curriculum. Faculty members who believe that PBL should be reserved for advanced students may be surprised to find that even their most senior students are awkward with the PBL process when they first attempt it. Gaining skills in working collaboratively, posing questions, developing and using effective inquiry strategies, and taking responsibility for learning are all processes that require practice and encouragement.

Educational programs that use PBL vary in their approach. Saarinen-Rahiika and Binkley (1998) described three general PBL models, including a completely integrated PBL curricula, a transitional curricula, and a single-course approach. The integrated model uses PBL as the primary learning method. The Occupational Therapy Program at McMaster University in Hamilton, Ontario, uses PBL, inquiry seminars, and skills labs in their second-degree, 2-year baccalaureate program (Royeen & Salvatori, 1997). A transitional curriculum uses more traditional approaches in the early phases of the program and then makes a gradual shift to PBL as students progress through the curriculum. The single-course approach encompasses implementing PBL in one or more courses across a curriculum.

The University of New Mexico (UNM) School of Medicine was one of the first medical schools to incorporate PBL into the curriculum. The UNM occupational therapy program uses a hybrid model that includes weekly PBL and the use of lecture, lab experiences, clinical fieldwork, and applied assignments. PBL has been built into the occupational therapy program since the program's inception in 1992. The program is currently an entry-level undergraduate one but will become an entry-level master's degree program in June 2000. Excluding Level II fieldwork, the curriculum consists of approximately 40% lecture, 40% experiential learning activities, 10% clinical education (Level I fieldwork), and 10% PBL. Beginning with the first summer session, students participate in PBL sessions for approximately 3 hr a week throughout their five-semester on-campus program. PBL is associated with one to three courses in any given semester. For example, during the spring semester of the second year, PBL is worked into the course

Applied Occupations III (Figure 1). At other times, PBL is woven into two or three courses across a semester.

Our experience at UNM, as well as our consultation with other occupational therapy educational programs throughout the United States and in other countries, has taught us that a program must successfully address numerous logistical challenges to obtain the benefits of PBL. Essential considerations include the need for small student groups, clear faculty roles and unified faculty attitudes, skilled and supported facilitators, independent student learning time, available learning resources, well-written and current cases, thoughtful case and curriculum development, matching PBL with student evaluation, and integration of PBL outcomes into program evaluation. We will discuss each essential item and describe how the UNM occupational therapy program has addressed each area.

Need for Small Groups of Students

Barrows (1994) suggested that the ideal PBL group size is 5 to 7 students. Others recommend 6 to 10 students. Dividing occupational therapy classes into small groups can be a major challenge for large educational programs. Assuring enough facilitators and small group rooms becomes more difficult as the number of groups increases. McMaster University admits 60 students each year and divides students into groups of 6 to 7 students each (Royeen & Salvatori, 1997), with students meeting 5 hr each week in PBL sessions. At UNM, we divide a class of 24 students into three groups of 8 students. We randomly assign our students to groups and facilitators. During the five semesters of on-campus learning, no two groups are ever the same. Each group of students works together for a semester and then is randomly reassembled. This, in turn, changes group dynamics and allows new groups of students to learn from one another.

During each semester, we have six PBL groups (three first-year and three second-year student groups) on a weekly basis. With a bank of trained facilitators and an available assortment of small rooms, this number of small groups is manageable. Occasionally, groups choose to meet off campus. PBL requires many small rooms instead of one large lecture hall. Rooms also need blackboards or flipcharts so that students can visually organize and illustrate their discussions.

All students must participate in PBL discussions. Essential skills that facilitate group problem solving include consensus decision making, ability to dialogue, accomplishing tasks, maintaining a team, and conflict resolution (Peterson, 1998). Students must take responsibility for other roles such as scribe and timekeeper during PBL sessions. As students become increasingly familiar with PBL processes, they begin to assume more of the facilitator role, and during the second year on campus, students cofacilitate cases in pairs. Student feedback indicates that this learning opportunity gives students a whole new set of skills that they believe will be useful in professional activities, such as

SCHOOL OF MEDICINE / DEPARTMENT OF ORTHOPEDICS
OCCUPATIONAL THERAPY PROGRAM

CLASS SCHEDULE

Second Year Spring Semester

	MONDAY	TUESDAY	WEDNESDAY	THURSDAY	FRIDAY
8:00 am 8:30					
9:00 am 9:30	Independent Study Time I I	OCC TH 420 Applied Occupations III I	OCC TH 420 Applied Occupations III Problem Based Learning	Independent Study Time I I	OCC TH 420 Applied Occupations III I
10:00 am 10:30	I I I	I I I	I I I	I I I	I I I
11:00 am 11:30	I I I	I I V	I I V	I I I	I I V
12:00 pm 12:30	I I V		Independent Study Time I I	I I V	Independent Study Time I I
1:00 pm 1:30	OCC TH 480 Organization & Administration	OCC TH 440 Community Health FWI	I I I	1:30 OCC TH 440	I I I
2:00 pm 2:30	I I I V	I I I	I I I	Community Health Seminars I I	I I I
3:00 pm 3:30	OCC TH 450 OT Assistive Technology I	I I I	I I I	V 3:30	I I I
4:00 pm 4:30	I I V	I I V	I I I	OCC TH 450 OT Assistive Technology I	I I V
5:00 pm 5:30			I I V	I V 5:30	

Figure 1. Class schedule.

leading team conferences. Students often comment that they never recognized how much work facilitating a group involves.

Clear Faculty Roles and Unified Faculty Attitudes

Although integrating PBL into the UNM occupational therapy curriculum was a relatively smooth process from the beginning, adding PBL to an existing program is often more difficult. Faculty attitudes can be a challenge. If a minority of faculty members value PBL, recruiting the support necessary to make PBL a reality may be difficult. One faculty member instituting PBL alone is almost impossible because that person would need to facilitate several groups working on the same case each week. Attempting to do so could be confusing and exhausting for the facilitator. Although all instructors do not need to be involved directly with PBL, faculty members need to support the spirit of PBL and reflect this to the students.

At UNM, five core faculty members all support each other in the PBL component of the curriculum. For example, a faculty member may write a case, facilitate weekly, or coordinate the PBL component for another faculty member's class. When PBL is part of a class, one person is assigned to coordinate PBL. This person may or may not be the primary instructor for the course. Coordination involves preparing and possibly writing new cases, securing facilitators, making and distributing appropriate copies of cases and feedback forms, meeting with all facilitators routinely, overseeing the midterm and final student feedback process, updating the case after the case has been completed, and providing troubleshooting among student groups. We have a faculty member who serves as a curriculum-wide PBL coordinator and is responsible for smooth integration of PBL across our curriculum. This person coordinates facilitator training sessions, makes sure that individual PBL course coordinators are aware of PBL details, develops and refines our feedback and evaluation system related to PBL, and coordinates the future directions of PBL. With permission from the students, this person may sit in with a group if a group functioning concern exists. We find that smooth integration of PBL requires cooperation among all of the faculty members and a willingness to assist each other.

Skilled and Supported Facilitators

Barrows (1994) stated that "the success or failure of a problem-based curriculum could easily rest on the preparation and training of tutors since their skills are central to the delivery of the curriculum" (p. 37). Saarinen-Rahiika and Binkley (1998) pointed out that faculty members must become facilitators of learning rather than givers of information. Shifting from a faculty-directed learning method like lectures to a student-directed learning method like PBL is often a major transition for faculty members because most of us learned to use more traditional teaching and learning methods. Wilkerson (1992) discussed two general facilitator skills. The first skill involves guiding the work of the student group and includes questioning and probing, encouraging critical appraisal, and balancing basic science and clinical emphases. The second skill involves promoting student interactions that support interpersonal relationships. Hitchcock and Anderson (1997) concluded that facilitators must establish ground rules for successful development of groups, deal with conflict directly as it arises, and intervene strategically to foster positive group development. Often, this involves observing student interactions and inserting thought-provoking statements at timely moments. New facilitators often comment to us that the biggest challenges were keeping their thoughts to themselves, avoiding giving the "correct" answer, and directing the conversation the way they thought it should go.

Training, support, and development of the facilitator is a high priority at UNM. By using the UNM School of Medicine model, we conduct 1½ day facilitator training workshop each year. New faculty members and community therapists who plan to facilitate in our curriculum attend this experiential workshop. Because we are a small group, we rely on community therapists to assist us in facilitating. After a short introduction to PBL, we quickly give the participants hands-on facilitator experience. By using a group of our students, the participants take turns facilitating the group for more than 6 hr. We use small rooms with one-way mirrors to allow the rest of the group to observe the session and discuss group dynamics and facilitator strategies. One experienced faculty member works with five to seven facilitator trainees. We run the student discussions for 2 days so that the facilitator trainees can observe the student group process and see how the group matures during a short period. The students return the second day with researched learning issues. We pay our students a small honorarium for their participation. In a classroom discussion, we cover such issues as the role of the facilitator, dealing with challenging situations like the dominating or quiet student, and the feedback process. We do not charge a fee for the facilitator participants but ask them to facilitate a student group in the future, which requires approximately 30 to 40 hr of volunteer time. We also give the participants continuing education credit.

After attending facilitator training, we try to arrange for the person to cofacilitate a group for a semester because we find that most persons need further support and role modeling from an experienced facilitator. Once a person is comfortable with the facilitator role, we provide ongoing support by meeting frequently with the other course facilitators throughout the semester. Details of the cases and challenging group situations are discussed. We require 15 facilitators each year and depend heavily on our trained community facilitators. The McMaster University program requires 60 facilitators per academic year and likewise draws from a pool of unpaid clinical faculty members or professional associates who contribute approximately 50 to 100 hr per year (Salvatori & Clayton, 1994). We have recently started paying our facilitators a small honorarium because we are finding that increasingly busy clinical environments make volunteering their time difficult for clinicians.

Advanced facilitator development is important for faculty member growth. Our medical school holds monthly "brown bag" PBL dialogues that are interdisciplinary. Participants suggest topics that have recently included strategies for working with quiet or dominating students, methods to give difficult feedback, and suggestions for assisting students to share learning issues effectively. Another method to refine facilitator skills is videotaping sessions and providing feedback to the facilitator.

Finally, students must be able to evaluate facilitator performance. The UNM occupational therapy program has a facilitator evaluation form for that purpose (see Appendix A). Similarly, Hay (1997a, 1997b) described an evaluation tool at McMaster University that provides written feedback from students to facilitators.

Independent Student Learning Time

If a program schedules extensive in-class time for students, then students may view PBL as an additional stressor. Time allocated for independent study is necessary to allow students to research learning issues on their own. To free up time, faculty members must determine which topics do not need to be addressed in more traditional lecture or laboratory formats. We find that when PBL is repetitive of material delivered elsewhere, the students are less motivated to learn. Our semester schedule at UNM always includes dedicated independent time for learning issue study (see Figure 1).

Available Learning Resources

Learning resources that our students use include the following: expertise of faculty members, community therapists, and other professionals; field trips; books (including textbooks); journals; the Internet; and anatomical models. When the UNM occupational therapy program was new, few occupational therapy resources were available in the health sciences library, and during our initial accreditation site visit, the students pointed this out to the reviewers. The students noticed the deficient resources because they were actively attempting to obtain various resources for PBL. From the first semester in the program, our students become active library users. They must purchase computers, and the librarians teach them how to conduct online searches. During tutorials, facilitators encourage students to use various resources and to critique the quality of materials that they bring to the group.

Well-Written and Current Cases

Good cases are central to PBL. Cases (sometimes called "problems" or "triggers") drive the learning process and are the trigger or catalyst that spark student interest and the "need to know." Cases come in many forms and can be creatively constructed (VanLeit, 1995). They provide some type of challenge for students and serve as the "surrogate teacher." According to Barrows and Kelsow (1996), successful cases should seem authentic (realistic), facilitate inquiry, approximate reality, and fit well into a curriculum.

Authenticity

Cases need to seem both realistic and relevant to students and instructors. In our experience, contrived or artificial cases tend bring about indifference or resistance. Students prefer to address challenges that are clearly the types of challenges that occupational therapists face.

Inquiry Facilitation

Cases must be presented in a manner that requires students to determine what else they need to know to proceed. If students receive too much information at the outset, then they are not stimulated to ask good questions and frame their own inquiry and analysis. In addition, the case format should never become too formulaic or predictable. If the students always expect cases to appear in a particular format, they may never develop the ability to handle unusual or unexpected challenges, or they may begin to believe that occupational therapy scenarios always present similarly in the clinic as well as in the classroom. The inquiry process may assist students to become comfortable with the ambiguity of occupational therapy practice. Students learn that no one correct answer or way of working through a scenario exists. The emphasis on informed and intelligent problem framing and problem solving begins to supplant the focus on "getting the right answer."

Reality Approximation

Students become excited by cases that seem real and move beyond paper. The use of videotapes, role-playing, practical experiences (e.g., actually attempting manual muscle testing in the context of a case), field trips to actual clinical settings, simulated or real clients, photographs, actual therapy equipment, and so forth all add a level of realism that is stimulating and facilitates enhanced learning (VanLeit, 1995). Students benefit from performing a task that flows naturally from the case, such as writing an intervention plan, progress note, or consultation report; demonstrating the use of adaptive equipment; or developing and running a group. Students find these activities to be meaningful and valuable when they are in the context of a particular case.

Curricular Match

PBL cases should reflect the expected knowledge and skill base of the curriculum. This means that cases presented early in the curriculum will probably be less complex than those presented later in the program. Cases may introduce new material, facilitate enhanced understanding, or stimulate integration of various types of information and skills. In addition, for PBL to be integrated successfully into a curriculum, students must consistently receive the message that student-centered problem solving, self-directed learning, and collaboration are valued. Otherwise, instructors may find that students become suspicious or resistant when asked to work in PBL groups.

Thoughtful Case and Curriculum Development

Case development becomes easier with experience. Initially, case development may take many hours, especially if several new cases are to be developed for a course. Case refinement continues throughout the lifetime of a case (which may be many years). Every time a case is used, the students and facilitators should identify what went well and what needs modification. Sometimes critical information is missing or inconsistent. Other times, practice changes and requires case modification. For example, one UNM occupational therapy case was about a woman who had a hip fracture and went to a rehabilitation hospital. During the years, shortening her length of stay and eventually sending her to a skilled nursing facility instead of a rehabilitation center became necessary to better reflect the realities of occupational therapy practice.

One must first determine the objectives for using PBL in a particular course before writing a case. Which aspect of a course best lends itself to PBL? For example, a case we used during the first year in a UNM occupational therapy physiology course was developed to facilitate student understanding of the physiological mechanisms that underlie the problems of persons with diabetes. The learning issues that arose were narrow and deep, and the case touched only incidentally on occupational therapy interventions. Much of the information students learned had never been presented before in any other format. In contrast, in a senior course emphasizing the psychosocial dimensions of occupational therapy practice, PBL serves an integrating function. Students have cases that require them to consider clients with physical as well as psychosocial issues and needs, and students must demonstrate the ability to evaluate and develop intervention plans targeting psychosocial needs. To work successfully through the cases, students must draw on information they learned previously in other courses (e.g., basic science, occupational therapy process information, theoretical frames of reference).

Faculty members must be familiar with the entire curriculum to write cases that facilitate activation and integration of previously covered information. The use of PBL requires that faculty members communicate with each other and develop a congruent and collaborative approach to curriculum development (Saarinen-Rahiika & Binkley, 1998). In addition, PBL is more effectively integrated into a curriculum when instructors are clear about the broader curricular intent of using PBL. In the UNM occupational therapy program, besides content knowledge, the curricular goals of using PBL are to facilitate student development of an interest in lifelong learning, clinical reasoning skills, effective communication skills, interest in self-evaluation and personal and professional growth, and appreciation for the diversity and complexity of occupational therapy practice. All faculty members using PBL in their courses must remember these overarching goals in addition to identifying specific objectives for the PBL cases that they develop.

Matching PBL With Student Evaluation

Students are sensitive to methods of evaluation. PBL will only work if methods of evaluating student performance are congruent with the goals of PBL. Our experience has been that attempting to use examinations to test material covered in PBL cases destroys the spirit of inquiry. Instead, students become focused on learning the "right" information, and they become angry and resentful at facilitators who will not tell them what they are "supposed to know" from the case. In addition, attempts to grade student performance with letter grades lead to tremendous anxiety and create efforts on the part of students to stand out in a group. This tends to have the effect of chilling students' willingness to reflect honestly on their own strengths and areas of concern, to explore what they do not understand about a case, and to work collaboratively. Instead, they become competitive and tense about admitting what they do not know. In essence, they behave in the manner in which they have learned to behave in the more traditional, competitive classroom environment.

At UNM, the PBL component of each course is graded as "credit" or "no credit," and "credit" is necessary to pass the course or courses. Students must self-evaluate at the midpoint and end of each semester by using the Student PBL Evaluation Form (see Appendix B). Students present their self-evaluation to their group (the facilitator as well as other group members), and the rest of the group then gives feedback to each person that may confirm, conflict with, or add to each one's self-critique. Each student comes to the group with areas of strength and areas of needed growth. The expectation is that each student will identify areas to work on and personal goals. Most groups of students begin identifying personal goals for growth on the basis of the evaluation form after the group has met only one or two times. Students ask for feedback from others, respond to suggestions and feedback, and regularly discuss how they are progressing on their goals throughout the semester. If they achieve a goal, then they set a new one. This process occurs consistently across the entire curriculum. By the end of the senior year, students have extensive experience in setting personal goals and in giving and receiving feedback from other students and facilitators.

The UNM occupational therapy program method allows for self-, peer , and facilitator evaluation of student professional behaviors and group skills, but it does not evaluate the competence of student problem-solving processes. McMaster University uses written problems, simulated clients, and oral "triple jump" examinations that require students to demonstrate their ability to pose questions, identify inquiry strategies, develop intervention plans for clients, and other competencies in PBL (Salvatori & Clayton, 1994). The London School of Occupational Therapy uses self-evaluation questionnaires at the end of each case to clarify learning objectives and to allow students to have an opportunity for self-evaluation (Sadlo, 1994).

Integration of PBL Outcomes Into Program Evaluation

The UNM occupational therapy program has implemented an ongoing system of evaluation and feedback concerning PBL. This system includes case, course, and curricular evaluations. At the end of each semester, a faculty member who was not involved in the courses with PBL leads a focus group with the students to discuss their perceptions of the strengths and concerns related to PBL. Students reflect on the strengths of the cases and what they learned, explore the amount of integration of knowledge that occurred, discuss the amount of time they were able to spend doing independent study, and discuss aspects of facilitation that they found useful or problematic. This information is compiled and discussed with the faculty members to refine or modify the PBL component of the curriculum.

We survey students about their perceptions of their education (PBL and all other components of the curriculum) immediately before they leave campus for Level II fieldwork experiences and again after they have been in occupational therapy practice for 6 months. They reflect on the usefulness of PBL in their educational preparation and in their success as occupational therapy practitioners. Students discuss the effect of PBL on their confidence and competence as clinical reasoners, professional communicators, and lifelong learners.

Making it Happen: Issues in Implementation

Although PBL has certain core features that set it apart from other learning methods, room for creativity and variability exists in how it is implemented. Watson and West (1996) described five occupational therapy programs around the world that all use PBL in individual ways. All of the programs believed that PBL is effective despite the fact that they integrated it differently into their respective curricula.

The cost of PBL versus traditional curricula is a consideration. In some medical schools, the costs associated with PBL are no greater than those in traditional schools with up to 100 students (Mennin & Martinez-Burrola, 1986). Other studies suggested greater costs associated with PBL (Albanese & Mitchell, 1993). Norman and Schmidt (1992) suggested that having students approach written problems individually or in small groups without a facilitator and then using faculty teachers for synthesis and explanation may be helpful.

Programs considering integration of PBL must confront potential institutional barriers to change. These include fear of loss of instructor control; comfort with the status quo; concern about educational innovation costs in terms of time, money, and resources; and sometimes facing a challenging system that values research and clinical service more than education (Kaufman et al., 1989).

Our own experience with PBL has been extremely positive. The key seems to be to start small; respond to faculty, facilitator, and student feedback on an ongoing basis; remain flexible; be open to experimentation; and keep it fun. ∎

References

Albanese, M. A., & Mitchell, S. (1993). Problem-based learning: A review of literature on its outcomes and implementation issues. *Academic Medicine, 68,* 52–79.

Barrows, H. S. (1994). *Practice-based learning: Problem-based learning applied to medical education.* Springfield, IL: Southern Illinois University School of Medicine.

Barrows, H., & Kelsow, A. (1996, May 19–24). *Problem-based learning: Problem design and curriculum development.* Presentation given in Santa Fe, NM.

Hay, J. A. (1997a). Brief or New—An investigation of a tutor evaluation scale for formative purposes in a problem-based learning curriculum. *American Journal of Occupational Therapy, 51,* 140–143.

Hay, J. A. (1997b). Test–retest reliability of a tutor evaluation form used in a problem-based curriculum. *Canadian Journal of Occupational Therapy, 64,* 203–206.

Hitchcock, M. A., & Anderson, A. S. (1997). Dealing with dysfunctional tutorial groups. *Teaching and Learning in Medicine, 9,* 19–24.

Kaufman, A., Mennin, S., Waterman, R., Duban, S., Hansbarger, C., Silverblatt, H., Obenshain, S. S., Kantrowitz, M., Becker, T., Samet, J., & Wiese, W. (1989). The New Mexico experiment: Educational innovation and institutional change. *Academic Medicine, 64,* 285–294.

Margetson, D. (1996). Beginning with essentials: Why problem-based learning begins with problems. *Education for Health, 9,* 61–69.

Mennin, S. P., & Martinez-Burrola, N. (1986). The cost of problem-based versus traditional medical education. *Medical Education, 20,* 187–194.

Norman, G. R., & Schmidt, H. G. (1992). The psychological basis of problem-based learning: A review of the evidence. *Academic Medicine, 67,* 257–265.

Peterson, M. (1998). Skills to enhance problem-based learning [Online]. *Medical Education Online, 2.* (Available: www.utmb.edu/meo/)

Royeen, C. B., & Salvatori, P. (1997). Comparison of problem-based learning curricula in two occupational therapy programmes. *Canadian Journal of Occupational Therapy, 64,* 197–202.

Saarinen-Rahiika, H., & Binkley, J. M. (1998). Problem-based learning in physical therapy: A review of the literature and overview of the McMaster University experience. *Physical Therapy, 78,* 195–207.

Sadlo, G. (1994). Problem-based learning in the development of an occupational therapy curriculum: Part 2: The BSc at the London School of Occupational Therapy. *British Journal of Occupational Therapy, 57,* 79–83.

Salvatori, P., & Clayton, K. (1994). Problem-based learning in action. *OT Week, 8(40),* 24–25.

Shin, J. H., Haynes, R. B., & Johnston, M. E. (1993). Effect of problem-based, self-directed undergraduate education on lifelong learning. *Canadian Medical Association Journal, 148,* 969–976.

Stern, P. (1997). Student perceptions of a problem-based learning course. *American Journal of Occupational Therapy, 51,* 589–596.

VanLeit, B. (1995). Using the case method to develop clinical reasoning skills in problem-based learning. *American Journal of Occupational Therapy, 49,* 349–353.

Watson, D. E., & West, D. J. (1996). Using problem-based learning to improve educational outcomes. *Occupational Therapy International, 3,* 81–93.

Wilkerson, L. (1992, April). *Identification of skills for the problem-based tutor: Student and faculty perspectives.* Paper presented at the Annual Meeting of the American Educational Research Association, San Francisco, CA.

Appendix A

UNIVERSITY OF NEW MEXICO
Occupational Therapy Program

Student Evaluation of Facilitator

Student: _____   Midterm _____ Final _____
Facilitator: _____
Course: _____   Date: _____

Comment on each category using specific examples when possible:

Knowledge base - content learning:
Probes understanding of material to full extent. Challenges application to other situations. Requires students to relate learning issues to client issues and concerns.

Problem-Based Learning Process:
Encourages issue/problem identification, hypothesis formulation and hypothesis evaluation. Encourages multi-dimensional approach to client cases. Helps students identify focused learning issues.

Student-Centered Learning:
Respects students as peer group learners. Active participant in group discussions. Maintains a non-authoritarian role. Encourages student-to-student interactions and student leadership.

Group Skills:
Helps resolve group conflict. Models critical listening. Encourages effective presentation of material by students. Models effective ability to give and receive positive feedback and constructive criticism.

Use of Unit Resources:
Helps to identify specific resources (faculty, community professionals, etc.). Serves as a resource person when appropriate. Familiar with case.

Appendix B

UNIVERSITY OF NEW MEXICO
Occupational Therapy Program

Student PBL Performance Evaluation

Student: _____   Midterm _____   Final _____
Facilitator: _____
Course: _____   Date: _____

Student's Self Evaluation
Rate the following objectives as either **Satisfactory (S)** or **Unsatisfactory (U)**.
Justify the ratings with the use of comments and consideration of the criteria to be considered when determining the rating. As few as one unsatisfactory rating could result in an overall unsatisfactory rating of tutorial performance. Ultimately the final grading of satisfactory or unsatisfactory is the decision of the facilitator. However, students will be expected to provide peer and self evaluation in the form of descriptive comments.

Professional Practice		S	U
Knowledge and Learning: • builds on previous knowledge • applies information of relevant breadth & depth • demonstrates understanding of concepts & information	Comments		
Critical Thinking/Clinical Reasoning: • uses evidence and data to present reasoning • reasons with new and previously acquired information • applies theoretical concepts to specific cases			
Professional Growth and Development		S	U
Self Assessment: • identifies own strengths and areas of concern • identifies and implements plan for improvement • modifies behavior in response to feedback	Comments		
Self-Learning Skills: • formulates relevant, focused learning issues • uses a variety of current learning resources • critiques & questions resources utilized			
Professional Communication		S	U
Information Communication: • summarizes information succinctly • explains concepts clearly	Comments		
Interpersonal Communication: • initiates and facilitates group discussion • helps define group goals and direction • provides constructive feedback • sensitive to group needs			
Please turn over and complete back side			

(continued)

Appendix B (*continued*)

Student's Overall Self-Assessment	S	U
Comments (Strengths, Areas for Attention):		
Student Signature _____ Date _____		

Optional Facilitator Feedback
Comments (Strengths, Areas for Attention):
Facilitator Signature _____ Date _____

PROBLEM-BASED LEARNING AND CLINICAL REASONING

Outside of the Textbook: Improving Reasoning and Changing Attitudes About Mental Disabilities

Elizabeth Cara

Elizabeth Cara, MA, OTR, MFCC, is Assistant Professor, Department of Occupational Therapy, College of Sciences and Arts, San Jose State University, San Jose, California.

A psychosocial theory and application class at San Jose State University incorporates methods to practice interactive reasoning, to change stereotypical attitudes about mental illness, and to improve therapeutic readiness. This article explains the class and its methods, describes qualitative and quantitative data that measure the outcomes of this "client in the classroom" project, and lists practices for developing a similar program.

This article describes an innovative, experiential component of the psychosocial dysfunction theory and application class at San Jose State University (San Jose, CA). Qualitative and quantitative data have validated the effectiveness of the class in changing novice students' concepts of persons with mental disabilities and in facilitating clinical reasoning. A convergence of diverse information forms the foundation for this experiential laboratory in psychosocial dysfunction. Issues current in occupational therapy research, practice, and education include the use of applied research, attitude change, mental health practice, and clinical reasoning in education.

Rogers (1983) first focused attention on the ethics, science, and art of clinical reasoning. Since then, others have described clinical reasoning as involving several forms of thinking (Mattingly & Fleming, 1994). Therapists use different types of reasoning in day-to-day practice (Fleming, 1991). *Procedural reasoning* is a condition-focused problem-identification and problem-solving approach. *Interactive reasoning* is a form of reasoning that the therapist uses when he or she wants to understand the patient as a person (i.e., to understand the patient's point of view of her or his illness and how that illness affects present and future functioning). *Conditional reasoning* integrates the other two types and projects an imagined future condition or situation for the person in reconstructing a contextual life. *Pragmatic reasoning* (Schell & Cervero, 1993) is similar to conditional reasoning but additionally concerns the "personal context of the therapist" (p. 609).

Various models for teaching clinical reasoning exist in the occupational therapy literature (Schell, 1998). Most advocate using qualitative methods (Mattingly, 1991; Mattingly & Fleming, 1994; Peloquin, 1989, 1993; Rogers & Masagatani, 1982; Schwartz, 1991), although one emphasizes quantitative methods (Neistadt, 1987). Rogers and Masagatani (1982) used qualitative methods to study how occupational therapists select, synthesize, and use data to evaluate a patient's status. Peloquin (1989, 1993) focused on the art of practice and discussed literature as sustaining the art. Mattingly (1991) and Mattingly and Fleming (1994) described clinical reasoning as narrative and applied phenomenology. Mattingly and Fleming (1994) discussed a clinical study involving ethnographic and action research methods. Schwartz (1991) discussed the theme of multiple aspects of intelligence and stated implications for teaching and learning. Schwartz advocated for a "connected teaching" approach in which the instructor teaches not only to the logic of problem solving but also to the mode of interactive reasoning. This approach is one in which students learn problem solving and interactive reasoning in a way that integrates cognitive and emotional intelligence in a context of intersubjectivity (Crepeau, 1991; MacRae & Cara, 1998; Stolorow, 1994; Stolorow & Atwood, 1992, 1994). Neistadt (1987) designed a model for the classroom that emphasized the science of clinical reasoning that Rogers (1983) outlined. The model involves using persons with physical disabilities as group discussion leaders. Although Neistadt's project includes some subjective data, it focuses mainly on the clinical problem-solving approach. In addition, Neistadt's project focuses solely on the aspects of living with a physical disability. Although it includes persons with physical disabilities, her "clinic in the classroom" model provides a secure base for learning about persons with mental disabilities. Providing models of learning about persons with psychiatric disabilities is particularly important because of the severe and prevalent stereotypes about them ("Mental Health Stigma Persists," 1999). Persons with psychiatric disabilities consistently rank among the least favored client groups of occupational therapy students (Lyons & Hayes, 1993). These stereotypes influence students' attitudes toward working in the mental health sector and, at best, may result in a shortage of trained occupational therapists working in mental health care. At worst, negative attitudes may severely influence treatment. Therefore, occupational therapy faculty members must design curricula that attend to students' attitudes toward persons with psychiatric and other disabilities.

This article describes an educational module that incorporates a connected teaching approach by including a third person aside from the instructor and teacher in the classroom. The project adapts Neistadt's (1987) "clinic in the classroom" model; however, some aspects differ from that model. Persons with mental disabilities living in the community serve not as group discussion leaders but as participants that a group of occupational therapy students interviews. The guest speakers do not come to tell the students about their lives as if they are group leaders but agree to enter into an interview with the students and answer questions about their lives. The instructor does not structure the interview, and the class does not usually receive information about the guest speaker. The class instructor is present but does not participate in the interview process. Outcome measures initially included quantitative ones to evaluate procedural reasoning as in Neistadt's project, but the major focus later became qualitative methods to evaluate outcomes regarding interactive and pragmatic reasoning and changes in the students' beliefs, feelings, and attitudes.

Class Setting

At San Jose State University, the main psychosocial dysfunction course is "Theory and Application of Occupational Therapy in Psychosocial Dysfunction." This class typically consists of a lecture with 55 to 70 students and three or four experiential laboratories that are held for 2 hr weekly and divide the class into groups of 15 to 20 students each. The class and labs occur during the second of four semesters of classes before Level I fieldwork practicums begin the following semester. This may be a student's only psychosocial experience before fieldwork.

Students often begin the occupational therapy program by fearing persons with mental disabilities. These fears are indistinguishable from typical societal stereotypes about persons with mental disabilities, such as believing that persons with mental disabilities are violent and assaulting, out of control, psychotic, deranged, and unable to care for themselves. The following quote from a student journal is representative.

> Because I was so surprised at how "normal" Lee seemed, I feel like the experience of having him come into the class and allowing us to interview him was very valuable. When reading case studies, people do not get the full idea of what a patient is like. For example, when I read about Lee prior to his entering the room, I had an image of some psychotic person who would probably freak out during the interview. Instead, he is just a man who has some difficulties in some areas of his life who needs the help of psychiatrists and medications.

Students' comments often imply a distance or separateness from persons with mental disabilities such that one can infer an "us versus them" attitude. For example, students are sure that "they" (persons with mental disabilities) are easily spotted and that "they" are different from the students or anyone that the students know in their lives. Students objectify persons with mental disabilities and tend to dehumanize them, albeit with much guilt, in keeping with media stereotypes and general societal attitudes.

Concurrently, students voice an inability to abstract and conceptualize about this population. A typical complaint is that students are unable to visualize the person or attach information they are learning to an image or a real person. They have many occupational therapy concepts in their heads but are unable to define the images clearly or to anchor them to real people. Therefore, I redesigned this experiential component to address the problematic attitudes and distance that students experience regarding persons with mental illnesses. The ultimate goal of this project was to improve students' readiness for psychosocial practicums by having students encounter a real person with a mental illness rather than relying on textbook descriptions. The objectives were to improve clinical reasoning and to foster a self-reflective, analytical, personal style of learning.

Redesigned Laboratory Procedures

Persons with mental disabilities who are currently clients in the mental health system volunteer to be interviewed as a group in each of three laboratories and are paid the current honorarium rate for guest lecturers (see Appendix A). These persons typically have schizophrenia, major depression, or bipolar disorder. Some have personality disorders and additional problems such as substance abuse, sexual abuse, or chronic physical conditions. They attend the lab for approximately 1 hr in which the lab students interview them as a group with the instructor present. Before the interview, the speaker signs a consent form and invoice, and the instructor fully briefs the speaker about the class and procedures in private. At the same time, the students discuss what information they will elicit. Both the speaker and students are aware of the interview format: The instructor introduces the speaker, the students introduce themselves, and the interview begins. The interview is an unstructured process in which students may not take notes (so that they do not disrupt their attention to the process). Both students and speakers know that the guest may decline to answer any questions or terminate the process whenever the speaker wishes. The instructor does not participate in the interview, which lasts from a half hour to an hour. The instructor debriefs the speaker at the end of the interview in a separate office. The lab after the first interview is reserved for a clinical reasoning session with the instructor and students.

When evaluating this project, the instructor experimented with two lab designs. The first design confirmed that procedural reasoning occurred, but this design likewise indicated areas for improvement. In the first design, before the guest's arrival, students read a case history of the guest's background and present functioning. Then the students made a list of problems and goals and a simple plan of treatment. They handed these materials to the instructor before the interview. The interview commenced in the manner discussed previously. After the guest left, the students wrote another list of problems and goals and a new plan, and the instructor assigned them to write a journal about the experience. The instructor, an experienced occupational therapist, compared the pre- and postinterview lists. An independent evaluator (another occupational therapist experienced in psychosocial dysfunction) additionally compared the pre- and postinterview lists.

The first design indicated that procedural reasoning did improve after interviewing a guest speaker. The students recognized problems pertinent to occupational therapy after the interview that they had not even noticed in the preinterview test. Additionally, after the interview, students were able to prioritize problems so that problems that demanded immediate attention and were more pressing received more emphasis. During the second lab interview, the postinterview list included problems that were not on the preinterview list.

Apparently, after the clinical reasoning practice, students were able to address problems implicitly. Recognition, prioritizing, and implicitly addressing problems indicated that procedural reasoning occurred.

Because of the frequency of positive comments in the students' journals about the guest speakers' influence on their attitudes and thinking, the instructor made changes to the second design. The changes included more guest speakers, a decrease in the time that elapsed between the guest speaker labs, and a focus on the content of the journals. Students now interview guest speakers in three labs during a 4-week period with the clinical reasoning practice occurring between the first and second labs. The instructor eliminated the pre- and post-interview problems, goals, and plan lists and now measures outcomes from the qualitative content of the journals.

In the second design of the lab, while the instructor and the guest speaker debrief, the students discuss the interview and use a data organization tool (DOT) to note their observations. The DOT is a simple tool formatted in three columns that asks for information, strengths, and problem areas that students observed. When the instructor returns for the duration of the lab, students and instructor discuss the process and reflect on the interview, students' observations regarding themselves, their behavior as interviewers, the speaker, or mental health in general. The instructor clarifies the assignment for that experience, which is to "write a minimum one-page journal of your thoughts and feelings about this experience, about your or your classmates' behavior, about the guest speaker, about mental illness, or about the mental health system in general." The instructor reminds the students about the confidential nature of the interview. In the second meeting, the instructor leads the clinical reasoning practice that is a treatment planning session by asking students questions about their experiences. The instructor distills the answers into broad categories of occupational performance areas and components. This clinical reasoning session often begins with students recalling observations they wrote on the DOT as the instructor encourages them to connect their information to the treatment planning categories. The session expands with the instructor's use of Socratic questioning, which encourages students to discuss and problem solve with one another and to analyze their own thoughts and feelings as a way of understanding the guest speaker and the intersubjective process (Crepeau, 1991; Stolorow & Atwood, 1992, 1994). At the end of the lab, students have formulated a beginning individual plan of strengths, weaknesses, and goals from understanding the guest speaker and the interview process. The hypothetical plan includes information regarding occupational performance that one can view from various models of practice.

The class interviews different guest speakers in a manner similar to the first lab during the next two lab sessions. The instructor likewise assigns journals for these two lab sessions. The instructor comments on the journals and returns them to the students within 1 week. Comments typically validate students' thoughts and feelings, motivate them to further action in the next interviews, ask questions to further expand thinking, or praise particularly astute thoughts and profound, genuine feelings. Eventually, students receive an assignment to write a complete, hypothetical treatment plan on the basis of their contact with one of the speakers. Thus, the assignment synthesizes the interview, journal, and reasoning practice.

The instructor used a qualitative method to measure the learning outcomes of this second design and carefully explored the content of the students' journals by using grounded theory (Glaser & Strauss, 1967). This qualitative method revealed outcomes of decreased stereotypes, increased self-understanding, improved attitude, affective change, and expanded clinical reasoning.

Three student assistants whom the class instructor had trained in grounded theory procedures analyzed journals for each session. Each assistant independently analyzed the journals' contents, linked themes, and established categories. The assistants then compared the analyses with one another to establish reliability. The three assistants noted and distilled common themes and categories in a dynamic process and constantly compared new material with previous content until saturation was reached. The instructor concurrently analyzed the journal content by using the same grounded, theory-constant comparative methods. The resulting themes and categories of assistants and instructor were further refined and compared. An independent auditor who is a colleague familiar with but not participating in the lab finally reviewed the content, categories, and themes to establish further trustworthiness.

Outcomes

The major category of comments analyzed from the journals concerned students' feelings about the guest lecturer and his or her life experiences. Common themes were empathy and compassion; insight and understanding of mental illness; admiration, respect, and appreciation for the speaker; and recognition of differences. Examples of empathy and compassion are the statements "Seeing a depressed individual was helpful to understand the magnitude of the illness," "I felt bad for him," "I can appreciate mental illness," "I wanted to help him, I felt sorry for him," " I enjoyed them," "sympathetic," and "really felt for them." The following statements demonstrated insight and understanding of mental illness: "I never understood before that depression could be so severe that a person could not perform ADLs," "made me realize that mental illness is beyond a person's control," and "helped me to understand so much more listening to someone with a disorder." The following statements are examples of admiration, respect, and appreciation for the speaker: "felt a sense of appreciation," "She was quite courageous to come," "appreciate his taking the time to come," and "surprised he was so willing to share parts of his life." The following statement showed awareness of difference: "It's hard for me to understand how a person could feel so helpless and hopeless."

The second most common category broadly concerned students' insights regarding the intersubjective personal process (i.e., awareness of themselves and their effect on the guest speaker and awareness of the speakers' influence on themselves and the interview). Common themes were awareness of the difficulty involved in the process, as exemplified by the statements "it was somewhat overwhelming," "I had a hard time with the interview," "entertaining, difficult, and challenging," "need more practice," and "wasn't sure how to ask a question." Examples indicating the awareness of the interview's effect on themselves are "I became quite drained watching her speak about her lack of energy," "amazed," "I was paralyzed during the whole session," "feel intimidated," "initially I felt threatened," "felt uneasy and pressured," and "made me nervous when he glanced up at the clock every few minutes."

A third category involved insight about the group process. Common themes were fear of other students' reactions and awareness of difference from peers, yet a sense of cohesiveness was likewise evident. The statements "intimidating to ask questions in front of peers" and "anxious about feeling incompetent in front of peers" exemplify the fear of other students' reactions. The statement of having a "group effort feeling" represents a sense of cohesiveness. The sense of cohesiveness was not superficial and indicated a mature group because students did not deny their reactions to other peers. They were frequently "frustrated by peers" or "bothered by other students' questions."

The fourth category indicates that the experience provided growth and learning. These were particularly common in the final journal assignments. Common themes were the worth of the project, the motivating and growth-stimulating nature of the project, wanting to know more, and growing confidence in ability and skills. The following statements demonstrate the worth of the project: "I feel these programs are a worthwhile cause," "great experience," "worthwhile," "interesting and incredible," "special learning experience," and "learned a lot about the interview process." Statements that attest to the growth-stimulating nature of the experience include the following: "in awe," "enlightening," "stimulating," "highly arousing," "challenging and thought provoking," "excellent adventure," "my ethnocentric views are lessening," "made me do a lot of thinking about people with mental illness," and "more beneficial than reading about it in a book."

Content revealed the motivating nature of the experience: "encouraged me to realize that [occupational therapy] makes a difference in the lives of the mentally ill," "want to do a better interview so that I could make a difference in my clients life," and "I want to know more." Evidence that the experience increased confidence and competence included "increased awareness of my verbal communication skills," "I was comfortable asking questions," "boost in self-confidence—I couldn't hurt or offend them," and "feel more confident."

A beneficial developmental progression during the three interviews was evident. The journal assignments from the first interview contained more comments about the difficulty of the interview and of the anxiety experienced. However, this self-consciousness and anxiety gave way during the second interview to learning about growth and the motivating force of the experience. The third and final interview included recognition of the positive effect of the experience, increased self-confidence, and direct recognition of changed perspectives about persons with mental disabilities. In all three sessions, most comments reflected a new understanding and respect for persons with mental disabilities. Many comments demonstrated the acquisition of a self-reflective ability with an awareness of personal feelings and knowledge of the importance of intersubjectivity in understanding the guest speaker and his or her own personal context. Overall, most students stated that this experience was a powerful force that changed their stereotypes and attitudes toward persons with mental illness and motivated them to make a difference in this area. Less expected, but no less powerful, was a growth in the ability to analyze the group process and to understand how the intersubjective process affected their thoughts and feelings about the guest speaker, themselves, and their attitudes regarding mental health. Thus, they developed a group and self-analytical ability that is critical to interactive, pragmatic, and conditional reasoning.

Conclusion

Opportunities for practicing psychosocial occupational therapy in a connected teaching classroom format (Schwartz, 1991) improved clinical reasoning and decreased stereotypes. Direct interaction with persons with mental disabilities improved problem identification and positively influenced attitudes toward a stereotyped group of persons. Pre- and postinterview problem lists demonstrated changes in procedural reasoning. Self-reflective, analytical journals demonstrated attitudinal change and facilitation of interactive and pragmatic reasoning. Merrill (1985) quoted Yerxa as "stating the need for balance between the collection of data that examine the efficacy of practice and data that contribute to theory on which practice is based" (p. 214). This project demonstrates the efficacy of educational practice, particularly in psychosocial dysfunction, on the basis of clinical reasoning theory.

Acknowledgments

The author acknowledges her students and the guest speakers who enthusiastically participated in this project. The Writing and Publishing Group of the Occupational Therapy Department at San Jose State University and Dr. Kay Schwartz graciously and thoughtfully reviewed earlier drafts of this article.

References

Crepeau, E. B. (1991). Achieving intersubjective understanding: Examples from an occupational therapy treatment session. *American Journal of Occupational Therapy, 44*, 1016–1024.

Fleming, M. (1991). The therapist with the three-track mind. *American Journal of Occupational Therapy, 45*, 1007–1015.

Glaser, B. G., & Strauss, A. L. (1967). *The discovery of grounded theory: Strategies for qualitative research.* Hawthorne, NY: Aldine.

Lyons, M., & Hayes, R. (1993). Student perceptions of persons with psychiatric and other disorders. *American Journal of Occupational Therapy, 47*, 541–550.

MacRae, A., & Cara, E. (1998). The occupational therapy process in mental health. In E. Cara & A. MacRae (Eds.), *Psychosocial occupational therapy in clinical practice* (pp. 3–31). Albany, NY: Delmar/ITP.

Mattingly, C. (1991). What is clinical reasoning? *American Journal of Occupational Therapy, 45*, 979–987.

Mattingly, C., & Fleming, M. H. (1994). *Clinical reasoning: Forms of inquiry in a therapeutic practice.* Philadelphia: F. A. Davis.

Mental health stigma persists. (1999, September 16). *OT Week*, 6.

Merrill, S. (1985). Qualitative methods in occupational therapy research: An application. *Occupational Therapy Journal of Research, 5*, 209–221.

Neistadt, M. (1987). Classroom as clinic: A model for teaching clinical reasoning in occupational therapy education. *American Journal of Occupational Therapy, 41*, 631–637.

Peloqin, S. (1989). Sustaining the art of practice in occupational therapy. *American Journal of Occupational Therapy, 43*, 219–226.

Peloquin, S. (1993). The depersonalization of patients: A profile gleaned from narratives. *American Journal of Occupational Therapy, 41*, 351–359.

Rogers, J. (1983). Clinical reasoning: The ethics, science, and art. *American Journal of Occupational Therapy, 37*, 601–616.

Rogers, J., & Masagatani, G. (1982). Clinical reasoning of occupational therapists during the initial assessment of physically disabled patients. *Occupational Therapy Journal of Research, 2*, 195–219.

Schell, B. A., & Cervero, R. M. (1993). Clinical reasoning in occupational therapy: An integrative review. *American Journal of Occupational Therapy, 47*, 605–610.

Schell, B. B. (1998). Clinical reasoning: The basis of practice. In M. L. Neistadt & E. B. Crepeau (Eds.), *Willard and Spackman's occupational therapy* (9th ed., pp. 90–100). Philadelphia: Lippincott.

Schwartz, K. (1991). Clinical reasoning and new ideas on intelligence: Implication for teaching and learning. *American Journal of Occupational Therapy, 45*, 1033–1037.

Stolorow, R. D. (1994). The intersubjective context of intrapsychic experience. In R. D. Stolorow, G. E. Atwood, & B. Brandchaft (Eds.), *The intersubjective perspective* (pp. 3–14). Northvale, NJ: Jason Aronson.

Stolorow, R. D., & Atwood, G. E. (1992). *Contexts of being: The intersubjective foundations of psychological life*. Hillsdale, NJ: Analytic Press.

Stolorow, R. D., & Atwood, G. E. (1994). Towards a science of human experience. In R. D. Stolorow, G. E. Atwood, & B. Brandchaft (Eds.), *The intersubjective perspective* (pp. 15–30). Northvale, NJ: Jason Aronson.

Appendix A

Essential Practices for Developing a Project

- *Informed consent and confidentiality:* Even though persons are hired voluntarily as guest lecturers, I ask them to sign a release-of-information form. They additionally sign a lecturer's payroll form and provide their Social Security number. At the same time, I explain exactly what will be happening in the group interview process, what they might expect, possible unanticipated questions, and that they are in control of this interview. For example, they can choose not to answer any questions and not to reveal any information as they choose. I additionally assure them that, although I have never needed to in the past, I will intervene if necessary. In other words, I assure them of their control and my support. I let speakers know that the students themselves are nervous. I express my gratitude for their willingness to participate. At the beginning and end of each group interview, I remind students of confidentiality expectations and responsibilities.

- *Payment:* Guest lecturers receive the typical guest lecturer fee, currently an honorarium of $25.00. This payment is essential; the one semester when I was unable to provide payment, some speakers did not show up as scheduled.

- *Department support:* Essential colleagues in my department agreed with me that the contribution of the guest speakers was invaluable and that no "professional" could duplicate it, so payment from departmental funds was not an issue. For those who were not sure whether they supported this idea, I engaged in an open dialogue and assumed responsibility for writing a policy for payment of guest speakers.

- *Grants:* Any grants possible can be helpful to pay speakers and for student assistance. A professional development grant ($1,200) supported the initial project and lecturer payment. Subsequent student assistance came from lottery funds ($600) (available for education in California) and from a small research grant ($300) from the College of Sciences and Art. All of the grants have different purposes. Some grants are available by modifying the project to fit different aims.

- *Student assistance:* Students are essential for the administrative work of outreach, contacting community organizations and speakers, transporting speakers, reminding speakers of appointments, and follow-up contact. Initially, I contacted persons I knew in community organizations and solicited their recommendations of who might be interested in the project. Then I contacted and interviewed patients. Student assistants were able to take over these tasks, including "cold calling" organizations. Local organizations were happy to ask their clients to participate, particularly organizations that emphasized vocational training. They viewed this group interview as excellent training for their clients. One assistant has been adequate for administrative details. Research assistants analyze data. When I have not had grant money available, I have worked with students completing independent study units or working on honors projects. I have asked specific persons to work with me; we then work out a quid pro quo contract that suits their needs and mine. Often students are eager to work with me in my class as a continuing learning experience in psychosocial dysfunction. Again, different ways exist to engage assistants.

- *Follow-up:* I believe that most persons want to make a difference; therefore, I make sure that I acknowledge their contributions. Students sign thank-you cards and formal thank-you letters on university letterhead stationery and send them to each guest lecturer and to the organization that encouraged them. Speakers often have recommended their friends; counselors often have recommended their peers.

PROBLEM-BASED LEARNING
AND CLINICAL REASONING

Brief Pilot Investigation: Evaluation of Clinical Reflection and Reasoning Before and After Workshop Intervention

Charlotte Brasic Royeen
Keli Mu
Kate Barrett
Aimee J. Luebben

Charlotte Brasic Royeen, PhD, OTR, is Associate Dean for Research and Professor, Keli Mu, PhD, is Instructor, and Kate Barrett, OTR, is Clinical Doctoral Student, Department of Occupational Therapy, School of Pharmacy and Allied Health Professions, Creighton University, Omaha, Nebraska. Aimee J. Luebben, EdD, OTR, is Associate Professor and Director, Programs in Occupational Therapy, School of Health Professions, University of Southern Indiana, Evansville, Indiana.

The current study reports on a preliminary, two-part research investigation regarding evaluation of clinical reflection and reasoning and the enhancement thereof. The first investigation involved 30 participants and examined the psychometric qualities of a questionnaire, the Self-Assessment of Clinical Reflection and Reasoning (SACRR), which evaluates the clinical reflection and reasoning skills of students and clinicians in occupational therapy and physical therapy. By using the SACRR, the second investigation explored the performance of 108 clinicians regarding clinical reflection and reasoning skills before and after they attended a 2-day workshop on clinical reasoning. The results of the investigations revealed that the SACRR had acceptable psychometric qualities. The internal consistency and test–retest reliability of the SACRR were moderate to high. A dependent t test revealed that compared with pretest scores, clinicians scored significantly higher (p = .00) on the posttest after attending the workshop. We discuss the findings of these pilot investigations regarding current educational and clinical practice in occupational therapy education. We also present the limitations of the study as well as directions for future research.

Clinical reasoning has been an area of increasing interest in many fields, especially in occupational therapy (Schell & Cervero, 1993). Rogers (1983), Rogers and Masagatani (1982), and Schön (1983) are among those who first directed the profession's interest to the topic. Clinical reasoning is the reflective thought process that therapists undergo to integrate client evaluation information and to develop and implement intervention plans. Furthermore, clinical reasoning is a central component in effective practice (Fleming, 1991a, 1991b; Neistadt, 1996; Rogers, 1983) and in education (Neistadt, 1987, 1996, 1998; Neistadt & Atkins, 1996; Neistadt, Wight, & Mulligan, 1998). A fundamental dimension of clinical reasoning is "reflection-in-action" (Dutton, 1995, p. 5). Critical reflection is "a way of thinking about occupational therapy practice in a manner that involves the ability to make rational choices and to assume responsibility for those choices" (Royeen, 1995, p. 338). According to Dewey (1933), reflective thinking is a self-initiated deliberation of beliefs and knowledge.

Researchers generally agree that the types of clinical reasoning in occupational therapy include narrative, procedural, interactive, conditional, and pragmatic reasoning (Fleming, 1991a; Mattingly & Fleming, 1994; Neistadt, 1996; Schell & Cervero, 1993). Researchers agree that novice and experienced clinicians maintain noticeably different clinical reasoning skills (Dutton, 1995). To teach students and novice clinicians to think like experienced or more expert occupational therapists, researchers and educators have begun to explore ways to teach and improve clinical reasoning skills (Neistadt, 1996; Royeen, 1995; Schwartz, 1991; VanLeit, 1995).

Although a great deal of literature on clinical reasoning exists, the majority of that literature focuses on "what is" and "how to" questions. Schell and Cervero (1993) summarized previous literature on clinical reasoning as "to either describe clinical reasoning or prescribe approaches to improve it" (p. 605). Clearly, research studies are necessary in other dimensions of clinical reasoning to gain a thorough understanding of it.

One area of notable omission is the development of ways to evaluate clinical reflection and reasoning. To evaluate the effectiveness of different teaching strategies for clinical reflection and reasoning, we need various ways to measure and evaluate the development and improvement of clinical reasoning skills. Currently, no quantitative assessment of clinical reflection or clinical reasoning in occupational therapy exists.

The current investigation consisted of two studies. First, we discuss a psychometric validation of a Likert questionnaire to evaluate clinical reflection and reasoning in occupational therapy and physical therapy. Second, by using the validated questionnaire, we discuss an investigation of the pretest and posttest performance of clinicians after an intervention (an in-service workshop on school-based clinical reflection and reasoning for therapists).

Instrument Development

Because clinical reasoning is grounded in the reflective process, we can evaluate reflection and the process thereof as a fundamental dimension of clinical reasoning. Roth (1989) identified that reflection is a result of the process of inquiry. He further summarized and operationalized the reflective process as a hierarchical compilation of 24 behaviors or actions. This compilation served as the domain specification of the instrument. Items for the Self-Assessment of Clinical Reflection and Reasoning (SACRR) were adapted from the list of descriptors that Roth postulated as critical reflection, or what we believe to be clinical reflection and reasoning. In this manner, the construct validity of the instrument was assumed because it was based on "detailed trait or construct definitions" (Anastasi, 1988, p. 162).

Second, the adapted questionnaire was informally pilot tested in various continuing education settings during a 2-year period before these investigations. The SACRR items' worth or value in evaluating clinical reflection and reasoning were solicited from practicing clinicians from across the United States and ranged from "very valuable" to "difficult to quantify." Thus, the validity check on item content or construct validity was adapted to include participant review, which is a type of validity check more common to qualitative methods (i.e., catalytic validity) (Grbich, 1999).

The SACRR consists of three sections. The first section addresses demographic information. The second section contains 26 close-ended questions that evaluate different aspects of clinical reflection and reasoning. These questions use a 5-point Likert scale from "strongly agree" (5) to "strongly disagree" (1). In the third section, respondents provide their comments.

Study One: Investigation of Reliability

Participants

Participants in the reliability study were 30 first-semester students enrolled in a bachelor of science of occupational therapy (BSOT) program at a Midwestern university. Three of the 30 participants already had bachelor's degrees at the time of the study, and the remaining 27 were working on their first bachelor's degrees. Age categories and frequency counts were as follows: 20 to 24 years of age, 18 participants; 25 to 29 years of age, 3 participants; 30 to 34 years of age, 0 participants; 35 to 39 years of age, 3 participants; and 40 to 44 years of age, 3 participants.

Procedure

During the fall semester, the director of the BSOT program administered the SACRR (pretest) and again 1 week later (posttest). Participants completed the SACRR in a group setting and took approximately 10 min to complete the instrument.

Data Analysis

Summated scores on the SACRR were analyzed by using the Statistical Package for the Social Sciences (SPSS) for Windows (1997). Internal consistency as measured by Cronbach's alpha further evaluated test validity (Anastasi, 1988). Test–retest reliability was examined by using a Spearman rank order correlation (Portney & Watkins, 1993).

Results and Conclusion

Cronbach's alpha was .87 for the pretest and .92 for the posttest, which suggests that the SACRR has high internal consistency (Bensen & Clark, 1982). The high internal consistency of the SACRR suggests that it is indeed measuring a unified concept and that the instrument does so in a theoretically sound and reliable manner. The Spearman rank order correlation coefficient (rho) of test–retest reliability was an "accepted value" of .60 (Benson & Clark, 1982, p. 796). Thus, the SACRR had acceptable psychometric qualities for pilot investigation.

Study Two: Study of Clinical Reasoning by Using the SACRR

Participants
Participants in this study were therapists who were self-selected to attend a 2-day workshop on clinical reasoning that the Florida Department of Education sponsored. Sixty-five occupational therapists, 19 physical therapists, 13 occupational therapy assistants, and 12 other professionals (special educators, nontechnical aides, etc.) attended and completed the SACRR workshop. Age categories and frequency counts were as follows: 20 to 24 years of age, 6 participants; 25 to 29 years of age, 17 participants; 30 to 34 years of age, 29 participants; 35 to 39 years of age, 22 participants; 40 to 44 years of age, 10 participants; 45 to 49 years of age, 19 participants; 50 to 54 years of age, 4 participants; and 55 years of age or more, 2 participants.

Procedure
The first author presented the 2-day workshop in December 1998 in Orlando, Florida. At the beginning of the workshop, participants completed the SACRR. For the final evaluation of the workshop, participants again completed the SACRR. The 2-day workshop consisted of 16 hr of didactic presentation, laboratory, and discussion about experiences.

Data Analysis
A dependent t test examined whether a significant difference existed between pretest and posttest scores on the SACRR. SPSS for Windows was used in data analysis, with the alpha set at .05.

Results and Conclusion
The results of the dependent t test revealed a significant difference between pretest and posttest scores on the SACRR (t [108] = 3.797, p = .000). Participants scored significantly higher on the posttest than on the pretest (106 vs. 101). These results suggest that intervention can enhance clinical reflection and reasoning (as measured by the SACRR). The results also suggest that an intervention using case-based instruction coupled with didactic instruction is an effective method for increasing clinical reflection and reasoning in therapists.

Discussion
Given the current focus on the importance of clinical reasoning in educational programs and clinical practice, various ways to examine and evaluate clinical reflection and reasoning skills should be available. A mixed-methods approach incorporating the SACRR (quantitative) as well as observation, interview, and journaling (qualitative) is probably the best way to evaluate clinical reflection and reasoning. The SACRR is not intended to be a stand-alone tool without addi-

tional data collection on clinical reasoning performance (preferably of a qualitative nature). Such mixed-methods performance evaluation of clinical reflection and reasoning can be useful in academic curricula and in continuing education. The SACRR can compare different instructional methods and educational activities for promoting clinical reasoning.

Future investigation into the reliability of self-report methodology when studying clinical reflection and reasoning is necessary to ensure the validity of the approach, with special attention to the potential threat to validity that choice of socially desirable items within response sets may create (Anastasi, 1988). Although the internal consistency of the SACRR is high, its test stability is moderate (Portney & Watkins, 1993). Further investigation of test stability of the SACRR is necessary. Future research should also examine whether differences exist in clinical reflection and reasoning between occupational therapists and physical therapists. Use caution in generalizing any of the findings of the current investigations to other sites and settings because the investigators based the sampling on convenience. ■

References

Anastasi, A. (1988). *Psychological testing* (6th ed.). New York: Macmillan.

Bensen, J., & Clark, F. (1982). A guide for instrument development and validation. *American Journal of Occupational Therapy, 36,* 789–800.

Dewey, J. (1933). *How we think*. Chicago: Henry Regency.

Dutton, R. (1995). *Clinical reasoning in physical disabilities.* Baltimore: Williams & Wilkins.

Fleming, M. H. (1991a). Clinical reasoning in medicine compared with clinical reasoning in occupational therapy. *American Journal of Occupational Therapy, 45,* 988–996.

Fleming, M. H. (1991b). The therapist with the three-track mind. *American Journal of Occupational Therapy, 45,* 1007–1014.

Grbich, C. (1999). *Qualitative research in health: An introduction* (2nd ed.). Thousand Oaks, CA: Sage.

Mattingly, C., & Fleming, M. H. (1994). *Clinical reasoning: Forms of inquiry in a therapeutic process.* Philadelphia: F. A. Davis.

Neistadt, M. E. (1987). Classroom as clinic: A model for teaching clinical reasoning in occupational therapy education. *American Journal of Occupational Therapy, 41,* 631–637.

Neistadt, M. E. (1996). Teaching strategies for development of clinical reasoning. *American Journal of Occupational Therapy, 50,* 676–684.

Neistadt, M. E. (1998). Teaching clinical reasoning as a thinking frame. *American Journal of Occupational Therapy, 52,* 221–229.

Neistadt, M. E., & Atkins, A. (1996). Analysis of the orthopedic content in an occupational therapy curriculum from a clinical reasoning perspective. *American Journal of Occupational Therapy, 50,* 669–675.

Neistadt, M. E., Wight, J., & Mulligan, S. E. (1998). Clinical reasoning case studies as teaching tools. *American Journal of Occupational Therapy, 52,* 125–132.

Portney, L., & Watkins, M. P. (1993). *Foundations of clinical research: Applications to practice.* Norwalk, CT: Appleton & Lange.

Rogers, J. C. (1983). Clinical reasoning: The ethics, science, and art, Eleanor Clarke Slagle lecture. *American Journal of Occupational Therapy, 37,* 601–616.

Rogers, J. C., & Masagatani, G. (1982). Clinical reasoning of occupational therapists during the initial assessment of physically disabled persons. *Occupational Therapy Journal of Research, 2,* 195–219.

Roth, R. (1989). Preparing the reflective practitioner: Transforming the apprentice through the dialectic. *Journal of Teacher Education, 40,* 31–35.

Royeen, C. B. (1995). A problem-based learning curriculum for occupational therapy education. *American Journal of Occupational Therapy, 49,* 338–346.

Schell, B. A., & Cervero, R. M. (1993). Clinical reasoning in occupational therapy: An integrative review. *American Journal of Occupational Therapy, 47,* 605–610.

Schön, D. A. (1983). *The reflective practitioner.* New York: Basic Books.

Schwartz, K. B. (1991). Clinical reasoning and new ideas on intelligence: Implications for teaching and learning. *American Journal of Occupational Therapy, 45,* 1033–1037.

SPSS for Windows [Computer software]. (1997). Chicago: SPSS.

VanLeit, B. (1995). Using the case method to develop clinical reasoning skills in problem-based learning. *American Journal of Occupational Therapy, 49,* 349–353.

Appendix A

Self-Assessment of Clinical Reflection and Reasoning (SACRR)

☐ Pretest
☐ Posttest

Demographic Data

Name: _____

Phone: (w) _____ (h) _____

Address: _____

Sex: ☐ Female ☐ Male

Please specify: Please check all that apply:
Age:
- ☐ 20–24
- ☐ 24–29
- ☐ 30–34
- ☐ 35–39
- ☐ 40–44
- ☐ 45–49
- ☐ 49–50
- ☐ 51–55
- ☐ 55 or more

Degree:
- ☐ COTA
- ☐ OTR
- ☐ MOT
- ☐ MSOT
- ☐ MS/MA in a field other than occupational therapy
- ☐ PhD
- ☐ EdD
- ☐ Other: _____

Response key: DS = strongly disagree, D = disagree, U = undecided, A = agree, SA = strongly agree

	SD	D	U	A	SA
1. I question how, what, and why I do things in practice.	☐	☐	☐	☐	☐
2. I ask myself and others questions as a way of learning.	☐	☐	☐	☐	☐
3. I don't make judgments until I have sufficient data.	☐	☐	☐	☐	☐
4. Prior to acting, I seek various solutions.	☐	☐	☐	☐	☐
5. Regarding the outcome of proposed interventions, I try to keep an open mind.	☐	☐	☐	☐	☐
6. I think in terms of comparing and contrasting information about a client's problems and proposed solutions to them.	☐	☐	☐	☐	☐
7. I look to theory for understanding a client's problems and proposed solutions to them.	☐	☐	☐	☐	☐
8. I look to frames of reference for planning my intervention strategy.	☐	☐	☐	☐	☐
9. I use theory to understand treatment techniques.	☐	☐	☐	☐	☐
10. I try to understand clinical problems by using a variety of frames of reference.	☐	☐	☐	☐	☐
11 When there is conflicting information about a clinical problem, I identify assumptions underlying the differing views.	☐	☐	☐	☐	☐
12. When planning intervention strategies, I ask "What if" for a variety of options.	☐	☐	☐	☐	☐
13. I ask for colleagues' ideas and viewpoints.	☐	☐	☐	☐	☐
14. I ask for the viewpoints of clients' family members.	☐	☐	☐	☐	☐
15. I cope well with change.	☐	☐	☐	☐	☐
16. I can function with uncertainty.	☐	☐	☐	☐	☐
17. I regularly hypothesize about the reasons for my clients' problems.	☐	☐	☐	☐	☐
18. I must validate clinical hypotheses through my own experience.	☐	☐	☐	☐	☐

	SD	D	U	A	SA
19. I clearly identify the clinical problems before planning intervention.	☐	☐	☐	☐	☐
20. I anticipate the sequence of events likely to result from planned intervention.	☐	☐	☐	☐	☐
21. Regarding a proposed intervention strategy, I think, "What makes it work?"	☐	☐	☐	☐	☐
22. Regarding a proposed intervention, I ask, "In what context would it work?"	☐	☐	☐	☐	☐
23. Regarding a particular intervention with a particular client, I determine whether it worked.	☐	☐	☐	☐	☐
24. I use clinical protocols for most of my treatment.	☐	☐	☐	☐	☐
25. I make decisions about practice based on my experience.	☐	☐	☐	☐	☐
26. I use theory to understand intervention strategies.	☐	☐	☐	☐	☐

From "Preparing the Reflective Practitioner: Transforming the Apprentice Through the Dialectic," by R. Roth, 1989, *Journal of Teacher Education, 40*, pp. 31–35. Copyright 1989 by Sage Publications. Readers can obtain a copy of this questionnaire from the first author.

ACADEMIC LEADERSHIP

Calls for Reform: A Conceptual Review of Educational Purpose in Occupational Therapy

Barb Hooper

Barb Hooper, MS, OTR, is Assistant Professor, Occupational Therapy Program, Grand Valley State University, Allendale, Michigan.

Given the complexities of a changing society and health care environment, educators have suggested that corresponding change is necessary within occupational therapy education. Consequently, a great deal of literature in recent years has concerned reforms for teaching and learning. However, no synthesis of this literature exists. This article reviews the academic teaching and learning literature within occupational therapy as it relates to educational reform. The article introduces the academic plan model as an effective way of synthesizing and evaluating the literature. By using the academic plan model, the literature falls into educational purpose, content, processes, sequence, learners, resources, and evaluation categories. The model is effective for examining areas of academic education that have been targeted for reform and areas that have received little attention.

Multiple factors both internal and external to the profession of occupational therapy have caused educators to reevaluate the curricular needs within the profession. Internal factors such as new knowledge, revised level of entry into the profession, and revised educational essentials for occupational therapy programs are driving curriculum revisions. In addition, external factors such as health care change, societal change, new knowledge paradigms, new technology, and new characteristics of learners have induced multiple reports of teaching and learning experiences, multiple descriptions of courses and programs, and some educational research within the occupational therapy literature. Therefore, as responses to internal and external change, the literature addressing occupational therapy education has included calls for educational or curricular reform.

Although much of the teaching and learning literature implicitly or explicitly promotes educational reforms in response to critical issues affecting occupational therapy, the literature has not been approached as a collective call for educational reform. Therefore, this article will review educational literature in occupational therapy as educational reform proposals. The review will draw from the academic teaching and learning literature published primarily in *The American Journal of Occupational Therapy* during the past 6 years and will highlight it as a collective call for reform. Certainly, work in the international journals would further illuminate issues affecting academic education. Including the teaching and learning articles from all of those sources, however, is beyond the scope of this article. Because of space constraints, the author did not include fieldwork education in this review. As an initial review, therefore, this piece will focus on one aspect of the educational literature—the teaching and learning of literature as it relates to reform within academic occupational therapy education in the United States.

In addition, because of the broad scope of the material, this article will use the academic plan model (Stark & Lattuca, 1997) as a framework for synthesizing academic teaching and learning literature as calls for reform. Using the academic plan model will help to identify the aspects of occupational therapy education that have been targeted for reform and the aspects of occupational therapy education that have received little or no attention regarding reform.

Overview of the Academic Plan Model

Practitioners in higher education developed the academic plan model to capture the comprehensive nature of the concept of "curriculum" (Stark & Lattuca, 1997). By using the academic plan model, educators constructed "a total blueprint" (Stark & Lattuca, 1997, p. 9) for curriculum design and evaluation that goes beyond the inclusion of "specific content or the use of specific instructional strategies" (p. 10). The academic plan model is a template that focuses conscious attention on a broad perspective of elements necessary for a strong educational plan. The elements to consider when designing a solid plan for learning include the following:

- The external, organizational, and internal influences on the program, the course, or the class
- Beliefs about the purpose of education
- The content or the subject matter
- The sequence in which the learner experiences the subject matter
- The learners for whom the plan is designed, their needs, what motivates them, and how they perceive the subject matter
- The instructional processes or the learning activities by which learning may be achieved
- The instructional resources, including materials and settings, in the learning process
- The evaluation strategies

The academic plan model is useful for designing and evaluating a single class, a single course, an entire program, or the curricular plan of the institution, all of which constitute a "curriculum" (Stark & Lattuca, 1997). Additionally, the model presupposes that any representation of curriculum (whether a single learning activity, a single class, a single course, the overall program, or the overall institution) embeds notions about educational purpose and content, instructional processes and sequence, learners, instructional resources, and evaluation (Stark & Lattuca, 1997). Therefore, the teaching and learning literature in occupational therapy, as a representation of curricular plans, embeds the elements of the academic plan model. This article will use the academic plan model, then, as a tool to analyze which elements of the plan the occupational therapy literature has considered and which it has not.

Although the elements of the academic plan are dialogical and not sequential, the authors of the model place educational purpose as the first element of the plan (Stark & Lattuca, 1997). The authors highlight educational purpose as the cornerstone of an academic plan because "the selection of knowledge, skills, and attitudes to be acquired reflects one's views about the purpose" (Stark & Lattuca, 1997, p. 12) of education. Therefore, this discussion will portray educational purpose as the cornerstone for the other elements and will organize the literature related to content, learning processes and resources, learners, sequence, and evaluation according to the educational purpose they reflect (Figure 1).

Educational purpose refers to the intended knowledge, skills, and attitudes that students learn throughout a program of study. The most common beliefs about educational purpose that faculty members in higher education hold include learning to think effectively by using observation skills, analytical skills, and synthesizing skills; learning to adapt to a changing society and to intervene in society to make the world a better place; learning knowledge and skills useful in a vocation that contributes to society's productivity; learning self-awareness and gaining personal autonomy; learning the great ideas of history; and learning to identify and clarify values (Stark & Lattuca, 1997). Although much of the occupational therapy teaching and learning literature overlooks an explicit discussion of intended educational purposes within the profession, the literature nevertheless implicitly promotes specific beliefs about educational purpose. This discussion will review the occupational therapy literature as supporting four educational purposes—effective thinking, societal change, vocational readiness, and the history of ideas—and the subelements related to each purpose. However, because different elements of the academic plan have received less attention in the occupational therapy literature, some purposes do not allow for discussion of all academic plan elements.

Education for Effective Thinking

Purpose

The most common, and the most explicit, call for reform related to educational purpose has been the call for increased emphasis on education for effective thinking. Effective thinking skills for occupational therapy graduates include both general intellectual capabilities and clinical thinking for job performance. General intellectual capacities include intellectual curiosity, knowledge organization, knowledge refinement, and reflective judgment (Royeen, 1995; Schemm, Corcoran, Kolodner, & Schaaf, 1993). Effective thinking for job performance includes thinking like an occupational therapist by using reflection and clinical reasoning (Neistadt, 1996, 1998; Neistadt, Wight, & Mulligan, 1998; Royeen,

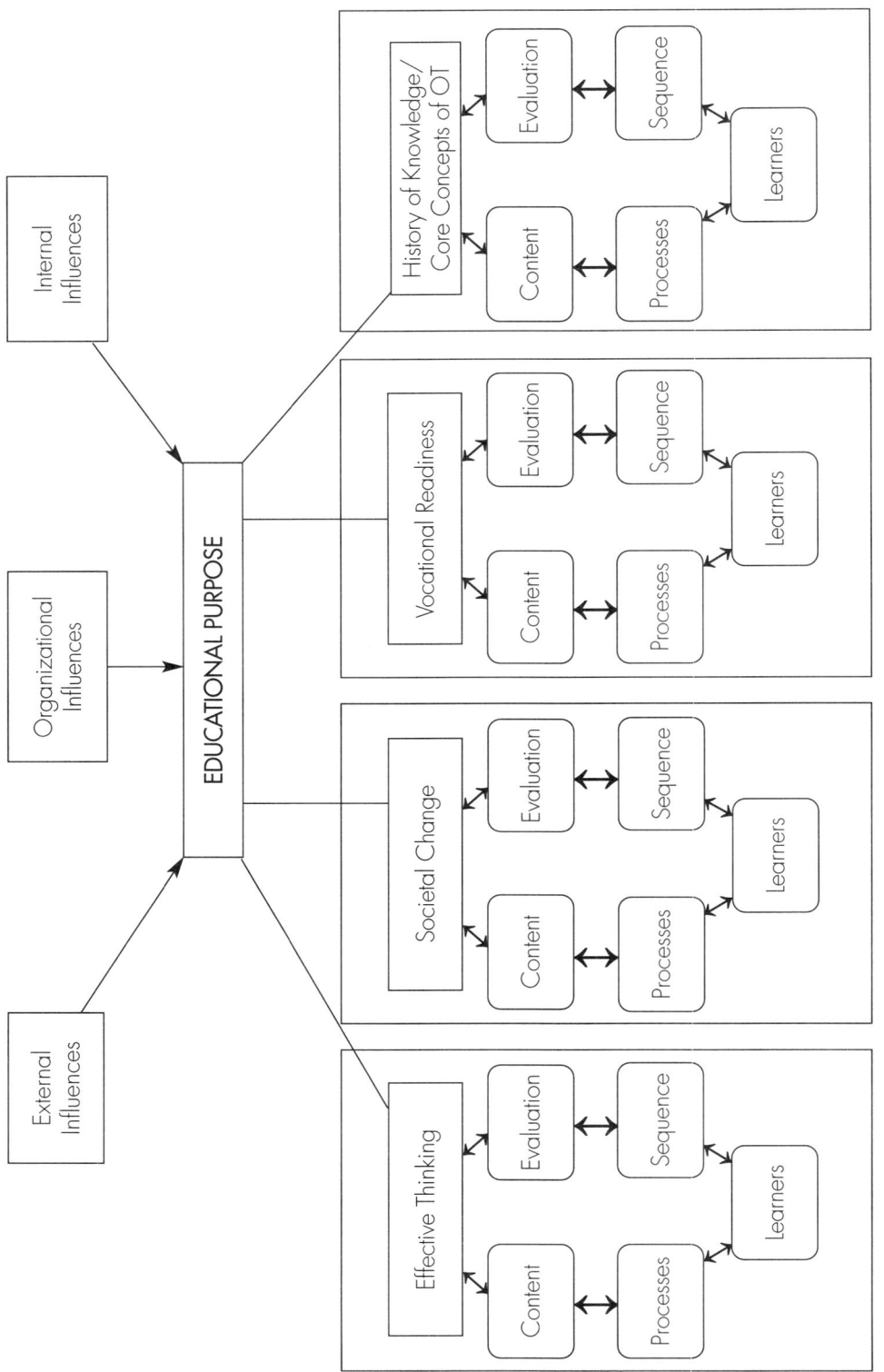

Figure 1. A conceptual approach to reforms for occupational therapy education.

1995). Thinking like a clinician involves the ability to consider the narrative, interactive, procedural, pragmatic, and ethical components of a case simultaneously (Neistadt, 1998; Neistadt et al., 1998; Schell & Cervero, 1993).

Content

Although educators promote reforms in educational purpose that will achieve effective thinking, most of the literature regarding educational content has addressed effective thinking for job performance more than it has addressed effective thinking related to general intellectual capacities. To achieve the educational goal of effective thinking for job performance, the literature promotes increased content related to clinical reasoning (Neistadt, 1996). Content related to clinical reasoning should have a balance between content focused on narrative reasoning and content focused on procedural reasoning within courses on adult physical disabilities. In one curriculum, psychosocial disabilities courses most often emphasized content related to narrative and interactive reasoning, and procedural reasoning was more associated with physical disabilities course work (Neistadt & Atkins, 1996). The imbalance indicated a potential procedural reasoning bias within the overall curriculum and within specific course content. Such content imbalance could cause students to miss important client information and to fail to address the rehabilitation goals important to the client. Therefore, to achieve the educational goal of effective thinking for job performance, clinical reasoning content must be balanced within individual assignments and individual courses and across the curriculum.

Learning Processes and Resources

Although clinical reasoning content has received considerable attention in the literature as an avenue toward effective thinking, specific content is not the primary focus of calls for more emphasis on effective thinking. In other words, promoters of effective thinking as the goal for occupational therapy education focus less on specific content and more on all content as a vehicle for developing skills in inquiry, critical analysis, reflective judgment, and clinical reasoning. Therefore, learning processes and types of learning experiences become as important as the content. Learning processes consistent with education for effective thinking have included problem-based learning (Royeen, 1995; Stern, 1997), case method (VanLeit, 1995), reflective journaling (Stern, 1997; Tryssenaar, 1995), classroom as clinic (Neistadt & Smith, 1997), and the clinical reasoning case study format (Neistadt, 1998; Neistadt et al., 1998).

Problem-based learning is a learning process linked to the development of reflective judgment, reflective practice and clinical reasoning, problem-solving skills, professional behavior, and learner confidence (Royeen, 1995; Stern, 1997; VanLeit, 1995). The classroom-as-clinic process (Neistadt, 1987, 1992; Neistadt & Smith, 1997) is an instructional method to help students learn diagnostic reasoning by completing classroom-based occupational therapy evaluations. This process has been an effective method for teaching diagnostic reasoning skills to occupational therapy students at the end of their professional academic course work (Neistadt, 1987) and during their first year of an entry-level master's program (Neistadt, 1992) as well as a method that may enhance diagnostic reasoning skills when using videotaped client evaluations (Neistadt & Smith, 1997). The process has been effective both in real client cases (Neistadt, 1987, 1992) and in some simulated cases (Neistadt & Smith, 1997).

In addition, one study in occupational therapy explored the use of interactive journaling as an instructional process that promotes self-reflection, which is a component of effective thinking. Self-reflection enables graduates to "deal with a profusion of changing skills and requirements" (Tryssenaar, 1995, p. 701). In a mental health module of 21 students, Tryssenaar (1995) found that journaling was effective in producing growth and development from an egocentric focus to self-awareness and an awareness of others.

Like educational purpose, authors have most often discussed learning resources in relation to effective thinking. Learning resources that facilitate effective thinking include paper cases, video cases, thinking frames, simulated cases, biographies and autobiographies, and journals (Neistadt, 1996; Neistadt et al., 1998; Tryssenaar, 1995; VanLeit, 1995).

Learners

The degree to which occupational therapy education is effective will depend on how well it interests and motivates the learners and connects with learners' previous experience and the degree to which learners are able to see its application to their future (Stark & Lattuca, 1997). The literature on education for effective thinking has primarily examined learner responses to processes such as problem-based learning experiences (Hammel et al., 1999; Stern, 1997; VanLeit, 1995) and clinical reasoning case studies (Neistadt, 1998; Neistadt et al., 1998). Few educators have addressed the diversity of learners in today's universities and how learner diversity affects designs for learning (Mitcham & O'Shea, 1994; Stark & Lattuca, 1997). However, most of the literature implies that learning for effective thinking requires learners who are actively engaged in the learning, share in the responsibility for their learning, and learn collaboratively.

Evaluation

Evaluation of learning within a paradigm of effective thinking has focused mostly on evaluating a few learning processes (Hay, 1997; Neistadt, 1998; Neistadt et al., 1998) for their effect on learners. Although these studies model scholarly evaluation of a single process or a single course, more effort is necessary to develop systematic evaluation and adjustment processes that specifically indicate learner development of effective thinking.

Educators have called for reform in educational purpose to move away from educating for entry-level skill and to move toward educating for effective thinking. In other words, curriculum design should focus on the intellectual skills to "engage in clinical reasoning" (Neistadt, 1996, p. 676), to solve problems that will expand future practice areas, and to create occupational therapy delivery models as societal values, demographics, and technology shift rapidly (Neistadt, 1996; Neistadt & Atkins, 1996; Royeen, 1995).

Because instructional process (and not content) is the priority within a paradigm of educating for effective thinking, discussions about content that supports the development of effective thinking have been limited to clinical reasoning content. However, instructional processes that promote effective thinking have received broader attention. These include problem-based learning, the case method, the classroom-as-clinic process, and reflective journaling. With the exception of learner perception and experience with key processes, learners and learning sequence have been overlooked as a focus in effective thinking. Some have addressed evaluation of a few learning processes, but this is most often limited to descriptions of a single course, a single program, or a single group's experiences. Little work has related to instructional resources that promote effective thinking, the developmental needs of learners for effective thinking, faculty competencies for promoting effective thinking, or the sequence of experiences for developing effective thinking.

Education for Societal Change

Purpose

Although less explicit than the reforms related to effective thinking, other occupational therapy educators have called for reforms in educational purpose related to societal change (Lyons, 1997; Lyons & Hayes, 1993; Lyons & Zivani, 1995; McColl, 1998). *Educating for societal change* refers to engaging students in contemporary societal issues to affect those issues through the graduates of the program. Therefore, teaching and learning focuses on exposure to societal issues, adapting to changes within society, identifying injustices, and working to intervene in societal issues (Stark & Lattuca, 1997). In occupational therapy, a few educators have linked teaching and learning approaches to social justice by focusing on the stereotypes that students maintain about persons with psychiatric disorders, even after completing their professional education (Lyons, 1997; Lyons & Hayes, 1993; Lyons & Ziviani, 1995). These studies suggested that education focused on impairments associated with conditions may do nothing "to dispel ignorance and fear" (Lyons & Ziviani, 1995, p. 1006). In fact, a focus on deficits in the classroom may actually perpetuate fear and pessimism about a group of persons with a disability. Although these studies explicitly focused on student attitudes toward persons with psychiatric disabilities, they implicitly proposed reform in educational purpose. In other words, occupational therapy education should consider ways in which it can promote a student's ability to fight stigma and oppression associated with disability, to advocate for persons whom society marginalizes, and to deal with professional and community attitudes toward persons who are disadvantaged.

Content

To help learners become persons who are concerned with social justice, educators must focus less on what to do and how to act and focus more on how to be a certain kind of person (Peloquin, 1995). For example, learning to be an empathetic person is quite different than learning communication skills that impart empathy. Therefore, if the purpose of education is societal change, then educators in occupational therapy must aim to facilitate learning in altruism, equality, freedom, justice, dignity, truth, and prudence (Peloquin, 1995). Content must move away from an impairment model (Lyons & Ziviani, 1995); however, the occupational therapy literature has not discussed specific content for helping students become concerned with issues of justice.

Learning Processes

Although the literature has not discussed specific content related to education for societal change, the literature has described a few learning processes that produce awareness, concern, and positive attitudes toward persons with disabilities. These processes include exposure early in the curriculum to positive information about persons with disabilities (Lee, Paterson, & Chan, 1994), exposure to clients outside of a medical model setting, exposure to client life stories (Lyons & Ziviani, 1995), and approaches to professional behavior that emphasize collaboration and power sharing versus detachment and professional distance (Lyons, 1997).

Learners

The most prevalent information about learners regarding education for societal change involves learners' perceptions of various client groups (Eberhardt & Mayberry, 1995; Lee et al., 1994; Lyons, 1997; Lyons & Hayes, 1993; Lyons & Ziviani, 1995). Learners in occupational therapy do not vary from non–health care students in their attitudes toward persons with mental illness. Likewise, practitioners are continually susceptible to prevailing stereotypes in society toward persons with disabilities (Lyons & Ziviani, 1995).

Sequence

Within the paradigm of education for societal change, only a few studies have considered the learning sequence. These studies suggested that learner attitudes may become more positive through information attained early in the curriculum (Lee et al., 1994; Lyons & Hayes, 1993). Increased amount of time spent in professional education was not linked to more positive attitudes.

Education for Vocational Readiness

Purpose

In contrast with education that helps learners to become a certain kind of person, some literature has emphasized education that helps learners to know what to do as an occupational therapist. Education as preparation for job performance focuses on knowledge and skills that will enable students to earn a living and contribute to society (Stark & Lattuca, 1997). Therefore, the role of the professional program is to help students reach their vocational goals. The occupational therapy literature during the past 6 years has not emphasized learning to perform skills to earn a living as much as it has emphasized learning to develop qualities essential for today's challenges. However, a vocational skills focus was implicit in some survey literature, most of which was published before 1993.

Content

Surveys have studied the prevalence of technical content necessary for learners to practice in specific settings. For example, surveys have explored the technical skills and content necessary to work in the school setting (Powell, 1994), with persons with HIV and AIDS (DeGraff & Bennett, 1995), and with older adults (Breines, 1992; Goldstein & Runyon, 1993; Stone & Mertens, 1991); to use biofeedback (King, 1992), technology (Kanny, Anson, & Smith, 1991; Marshall, 1991), and crafts (Dickerson & Kaplan, 1991); to teach independent living skills (Richards, 1995); and to provide students with job skills, such as time management (Powell, 1994).

Although the literature during the past 6 years has not emphasized technical skills as the primary aim for occupational therapy education, the interpersonal aspects of job performance have received some attention. For example, in one curriculum, faculty members were concerned that students have opportunities for learning and practicing self-awareness and interpersonal competence. Fidler (1996) described professional behaviors that graduates need for competent practice. The professional behaviors of positive self-regard, increased self-awareness, interpersonal competence, and a commitment to learning were included, along with very specific behaviors that helped to operationalize professional behavior for faculty members and for learners.

Learning Processes

In addition to the behavioral approach to learning interpersonal skills, Peloquin and Babola analyzed the interpersonal aspects of practice as they occur in the clinical environment (Babola & Peloquin, 1999; Peloquin & Babola, 1996). After identifying key abilities necessary for competent clinical practice, including the ability to respond to unexpected events, to think "on the spot," to express ideas clearly, to listen actively and to respond to colleagues, to tolerate ambiguity, to give clear feedback, and to invite healthy debate, the authors designed learning processes for the classroom that gave learners the opportunity to develop these skills before entering the clinic.

Education Related to the History of Knowledge and Core Professional Concepts

Purpose

Although educational beliefs related to effective thinking, societal change, and vocational readiness were prevalent in occupational therapy before 1997, more recently, educational reforms have focused on the history and core philosophy of the profession, namely the role of occupation in health (Fisher, 1998; Nielson, 1998; Wood, 1998; Yerxa, 1995, 1998a, 1998b). The conceptual history and core beliefs of occupational therapy must be explicit in each course and in the overall curriculum. These educators believe that "the design of entry-level education is more than an organizational plan for making students learn facts and skills; it is the faculty's image of future practice" (Schemm et al., 1993, p. 626). Essentially, these authors call for reform in how academic programs view their role in practice. They recommend that education programs design a curriculum in ways that produce graduates who will lead and change practice and who can "articulately translate occupation into meaningful therapy programs" (Nielson, 1998, p. 386). Such a curriculum would centralize the idea of occupation, differentiate occupational therapy from other disciplines, balance medical knowledge with the study of occupation, and make occupation the focus of scholarly work (Yerxa, 1998b).

Although these educators promote education and research that centralizes the study of occupation, their reform proposals are closely linked to education for effective thinking and education for societal change. In other words, these educators propose that curricular design that explicitly makes occupation the subject of study will allow learners to use occupation as their framework for thinking effectively about occupational therapy intervention. Furthermore, a curriculum with occupation as the core organizing principle will produce graduates who will "exert a stronger and more positive impact on society as a whole" (Yerxa, 1998b, p. 371).

Content and Learning Processes

Within the paradigm of education organized around the great ideas of occupational therapy, content and scholarship related to occupation must be centralized. This content would include new knowledge about the human being as essentially occupational, about the dynamic between occupation and health, and about the relevance of occupation to wellness and disability. Apart from these broad core topics, specific content is at the discretion of each individual program. Each program should, however, adopt learning processes that give learners autonomy and self-direction (Yerxa, 1998b).

Discussion

The occupational therapy educational literature has responded to societal and professional change by proposing reforms for academic education. Educational reforms represent, whether implicitly or explicitly, notions of curriculum that include beliefs about the purpose of education, which in turn shapes strategies for content, learning processes and resources, learners, learning sequence, and evaluation of learning (see Figure 2).

New strategies for academic teaching and learning equip practitioners with the ability to manage the multifaceted principles, complexities, and ambiguities of practice. New teaching and learning strategies help students to develop the critical reflection that they will need to be successful in increasingly complex societal systems (Foto, 1997; Neistadt, 1996; Royeen, 1995; Schemm et al., 1993).

This article has proposed the academic plan model (Stark & Lattuca, 1997) as one way of synthesizing proposals related to teaching and learning. The academic plan model is a blueprint for understanding the dynamic elements that shape strong plans for learning. The model is useful as an organizing framework for designing learning plans more effectively, for examining curricular issues, and for guiding educational research. In this article, the model has helped to illuminate several key points about the teaching and learning literature in occupational therapy:

- Educational reform has been a key theme throughout the recent teaching and learning literature.
- Approaches to reform fall into four educational purposes; however, all four overlap.
- Much of the discussion about educational purpose has remained implicit.
- Educational purpose and instructional processes have received more attention than the other elements of the academic plan.
- Much of the work regarding the elements of the academic plan has lacked a conceptual framework.

By using the academic plan model for analysis of the teaching and learning literature in occupational therapy, one can see that the literature during the past 6 years has consistently emphasized the need for reform in occupational therapy education (Foto, 1997; Neistadt, 1996; Royeen, 1995; Schemm et al., 1993; Yerxa, 1998b), but not all of the elements involved in strong curricular planning have received equal emphasis. Educators argue that traditional occupational therapy education, which focuses on entry-level skill mastery, is not sufficient for

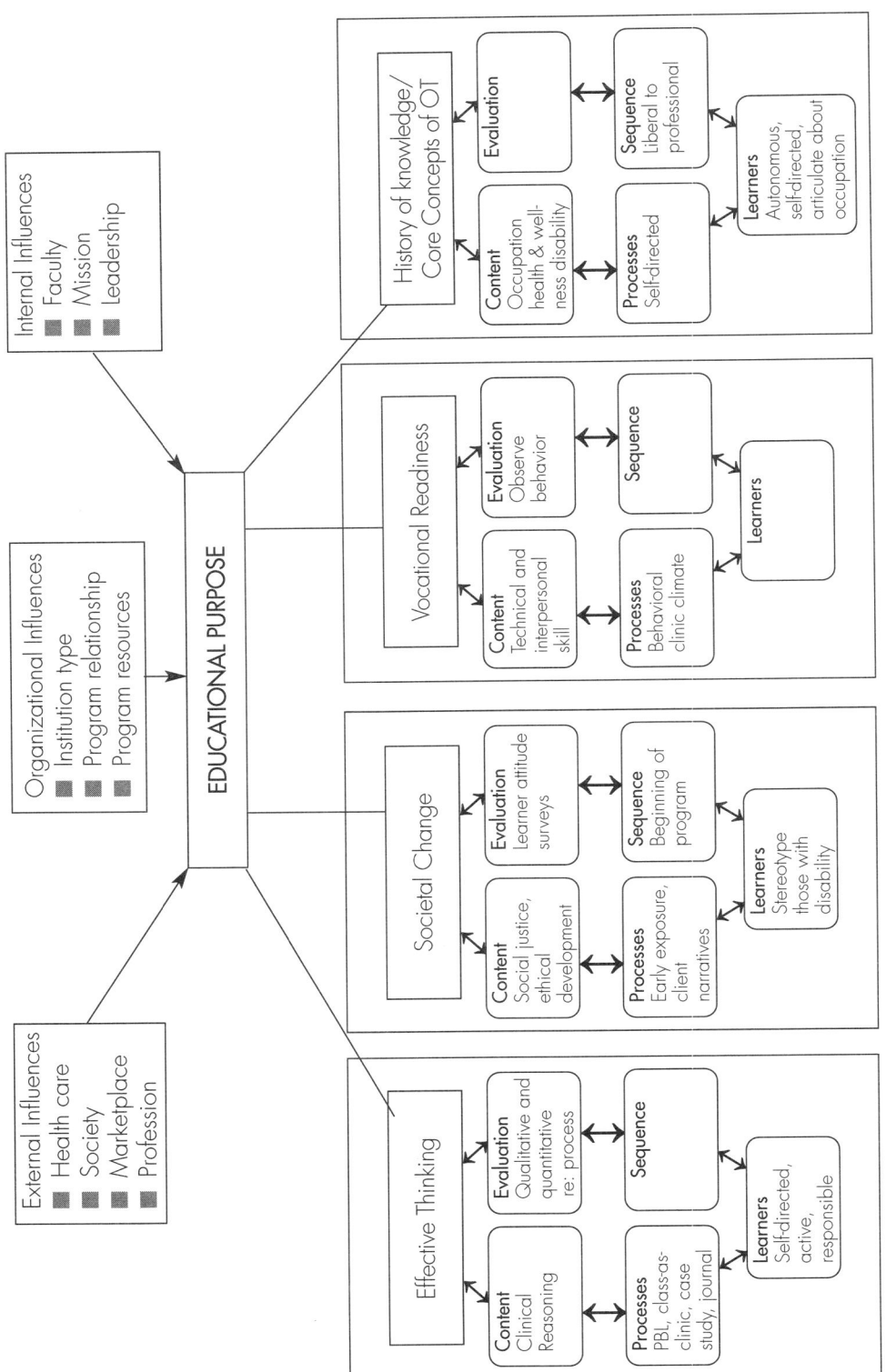

Figure 2. Current status of reform recommendations for occupational therapy education.

preparing graduates to meet the demands of health care and society in the 21st century (Foto, 1997; Neistadt, 1996; Royeen, 1995; Schemm et al., 1993; Yerxa, 1998b). However, educators have proposed different approaches for reform in occupational therapy education. Some have proposed reforms related to effective thinking, and others have focused on reforms leading to societal change, vocational readiness, and education designed around historical knowledge and new knowledge about human occupation.

Regardless of the specific approach to reform, overlap is evident among the four approaches. For example, educators who highlight effective thinking as central to occupational therapy often use vocational readiness as one rationale. In other words, to be prepared for shifting vocational settings and roles, learners need general intellectual capabilities involved in using reflective judgment. Additionally, in proposals concerned with occupation as the cornerstone for curricular reform, learners still require self-direction and autonomy, learners must develop concern for social justice for persons with disabilities, and learners must use the core knowledge of the profession to think effectively about practice and scholarship. Likewise, when highlighting social justice or change issues in occupational therapy education reform, one essential component learners must develop is critical reflection.

The discussion of educational purposes and how they overlap is important for several reasons. First, much of our emphasis on educational purpose has remained implicit, yet our reform proposals stem from strong convictions about occupational therapy education. Second, considering the purposes within our proposals for education can direct our attention to the assumptions of instructional processes, content, course sequences, and evaluation strategies. In addition, making educational purposes explicit can be helpful in intentionally and consistently selecting the other elements of the academic plan that are necessary for strong curricula.

Because educational purpose in the occupational therapy literature has remained primarily implicit, the literature has been more specific when discussing instructional processes. By highlighting the literature as proposals for change, one sees that instructional processes are not separate from curriculum reform, and instructional processes are not separate from educational purpose, but seldom are instructional processes discussed in tandem with educational reform or purpose.

Because educational purpose and instructional processes have received most of the emphasis in the occupational therapy teaching and learning literature, the remaining elements within the academic plan have received less attention. Although they are mentioned throughout the literature, content, sequence of the subject matter, the learners for whom the plan is designed, instructional resources, and evaluation strategies have not been the key subjects of written descriptions or scholarship related to occupational therapy education.

Much of the literature, however, whether addressing purpose, content, processes, learners, sequence, resources, or evaluation, does so outside of a conceptual framework (see Figure 2). In other words, the literature often addresses one topic, such as an instructional process, without linking it conceptually to educational purpose and to other elements of the academic plan model. Applying the academic plan as a framework for the teaching and learning literature illustrates that we have not used an integrated approach in our educational reform proposals. Consequently, the teaching and learning literature can seem sketchy and disconnected from a theoretical model. In addition to the need for integration, using the academic plan model for analysis and synthesis of the literature suggests the need for intentionality among all elements of a learning plan. In other words, a plan implies "both intentions and rational choices" (Stark & Lattuca, 1997, p. 9) among alternatives related to content, learning processes, sequences, resources, and evaluations. Much of the discussion about instructional processes indicates why one process was selected over dissimilar processes (e.g., problem-based learning vs. lecture), but little discussion has outlined why an instructional process was selected over similar processes.

Conclusion

The elements of the academic plan model can be useful in developing curriculum and learning activities, evaluating curriculum and learning activities, and guiding future curricular research. The model can be a blueprint for designing programs with intentionality and coherence among the academic plan elements. As an evaluation tool, the model can guide evaluation to consider elements of the academic plan that are not generally considered. As a guide for inquiry, the model can help to generate research questions related to specific elements of the academic plan. For example, more research is necessary regarding learner characteristics, content, resources, and learning sequences. These research questions should reflect many pedagogical perspectives, including critical and feminist pedagogy as well as performance-based pedagogies. In addition, research questions could emerge regarding relationships among the elements of the academic plan (e.g., the relationship between instructional processes and educational purpose), relationships among educational aims and evaluation strategies, and the effect of external and organizational influences on emerging occupational therapy academic plans. ■

References

Babola, K. A., & Peloquin, S. M. (1999). Making a clinical climate in the classroom: An assessment. *American Journal of Occupational Therapy, 53*, 373–380.

Breines, E. B. (1992). Preparing occupational therapy students for practice with the elderly. *Physical and Occupational Therapy in Geriatrics, 10*(3), 47–55.

DeGraff, M. S., & Bennett, D. (1995). Survey of HIV/AIDS related curricula in programs of occupational therapy. *Occupational Therapy in Health Care, 9*, 3–20.

Dickerson, A., & Kaplan, S. H. (1991). A comparison of craft use and academic preparation in craft modalities. *American Journal of Occupational Therapy, 45*, 11–17.

Eberhardt, K., & Mayberry, W. (1995). Factors influencing entry-level occupational therapists' attitudes toward persons with disabilities. *American Journal of Occupational Therapy, 49*, 629–636.

Fidler, G. S. (1996). Brief or New—Developing a repertoire of professional behaviors. *American Journal of Occupational Therapy, 50*, 583–587.

Fisher, A. G. (1998). Uniting practice and theory in an occupational framework, 1998 Eleanor Clarke Slagle lecture. *American Journal of Occupational Therapy, 52*, 509–522.

Foto, M. (1997). Nationally Speaking—Preparing occupational therapists for the year 2000: The impact of managed care on education and training. *American Journal of Occupational Therapy, 51*, 88–90.

Goldstein, H., & Runyon, C. (1993). An occupational therapy educational module to increase sensitivity about geriatric sexuality. *Physical and Occupational Therapy in Geriatrics, 11*, 57–76.

Hammel, J., Royeen, C. B., Bagatell, N., Chandler, B., Jensen, G., Loveland, J., & Stone, G. (1999). Student perspectives on problem-based learning in an occupational therapy curriculum: A multiyear qualitative evaluation. *American Journal of Occupational Therapy, 53*, 199–206.

Hay, J. A. (1997). Brief or New—An investigation of a tutor evaluation scale for formative purposes in a problem-based learning curriculum. *American Journal of Occupational Therapy, 50*, 140–143.

Kanny, E. M., Anson, D. K., & Smith, R. O. (1991). A survey of technology education in entry-level curricula: Quantity, quality, and barriers. *Occupational Therapy Journal of Research, 11*, 311–319.

King, T. I. (1992). Biofeedback: A survey regarding current clinical use and content in occupational therapy educational curricula. *Occupational Therapy Journal of Research, 12*, 50–58.

Lee, T. M. C., Paterson, J. G., & Chan, C. C. H. (1994). The effect of occupational therapy education on student's perceived attitudes toward persons with disabilities. *American Journal of Occupational Therapy, 48*, 633–638.

Lyons, M. (1997). Understanding professional behavior: Experiences of occupational therapy students in mental health settings. *American Journal of Occupational Therapy, 51*, 686–692.

Lyons, M., & Hayes, R. (1993). Student perceptions of persons with psychiatric and other disorders. *American Journal of Occupational Therapy, 47*, 541–548.

Lyons, M., & Ziviani, J. (1995). Stereotypes, stigma, and mental illness: Learning from fieldwork experiences. *American Journal of Occupational Therapy, 49*, 1002–1008.

Marshall, E. (1991). A survey of occupational therapy curricula. *American Journal of Occupational Therapy, 45,* 932–935.

McColl, M. A. (1998). What do we need to know in order to practice occupational therapy in the community? *American Journal of Occupational Therapy, 52,* 11–18.

Mitcham, M. D., & O'Shea, B. J. (1994). Using audioteleconferencing to link occupational therapy graduate students in the United States and Canada. *American Journal of Occupational Therapy, 48,* 619–625.

Neistadt, M. E. (1987). Classroom as clinic: A model for teaching clinical reasoning in occupational therapy education. *American Journal of Occupational Therapy, 41,* 631–637.

Neistadt, M. E. (1992). The classroom as clinic: Applications for a method of teaching clinical reasoning. *American Journal of Occupational Therapy, 46,* 814–819.

Neistadt, M. E. (1996). Teaching strategies for the development of clinical reasoning. *American Journal of Occupational Therapy, 50,* 676–684.

Neistadt, M. E. (1998). Teaching clinical reasoning as a thinking frame. *American Journal of Occupational Therapy, 52,* 221–230.

Neistadt, M. E., & Atkins, A. (1996). Analysis of the orthopedic content in an occupational therapy curriculum from a clinical reasoning perspective. *American Journal of Occupational Therapy, 50,* 669–675.

Neistadt, M. E., & Smith, R. E. (1997). Teaching diagnostic reasoning: Using a classroom-as-clinic methodology with videotapes. *American Journal of Occupational Therapy, 51,* 360–368.

Neistadt, M. E., Wight, J., & Mulligan, S. E. (1998). Clinical reasoning case studies as teaching tools. *American Journal of Occupational Therapy, 52,* 125–133.

Nielson, C. (1998). The Issue Is—How can academic culture move toward occupation-centered education? *American Journal of Occupational Therapy, 52,* 386–387.

Peloquin, S. M. (1995). The Issue Is—Communication skills: Why not turn to a skills training model? *American Journal of Occupational Therapy, 49,* 721–723.

Peloquin, S. M., & Babola, K. A. (1996). Brief or New—Making a clinical climate in the classroom. *American Journal of Occupational Therapy, 50,* 894–899.

Powell, N. J. (1994). Content for educational programs in school-based occupational therapy from a practice perspective. *American Journal of Occupational Therapy, 48,* 130–137.

Richards, L. (1995). Providing instruction in independent living and vocational rehabilitation for individuals with head injuries within an entry-level occupational therapy curriculum. *Occupational Therapy in Health Care, 9,* 57–70.

Royeen, C. B. (1995). A problem-based learning curriculum for occupational therapy education. *American Journal of Occupational Therapy, 49,* 338–346.

Schell, B. A., & Cervero, R. M. (1993). Clinical reasoning in occupational therapy: An integrative review. *American Journal of Occupational Therapy, 47,* 605–610.

Schemm, R. L., Corcoran, M., Kolodner, E., & Schaaf, R. (1993). A curriculum based on systems theory. *American Journal of Occupational Therapy, 47,* 625–634.

Stark, J. S., & Lattuca, L. R. (1997). *Shaping the college curriculum: Academic plans in action.* Boston: Allyn & Bacon.

Stern, P. (1997). Student perceptions of a problem-based learning course. *American Journal of Occupational Therapy, 51,* 589–596.

Stone, R. G., & Mertens, K. B. (1991). Educating entry-level occupational therapy students in gerontology. *American Journal of Occupational Therapy, 45,* 643–650.

Tryssenaar, J. (1995). Interactive journals: An educational strategy to promote reflection. *American Journal of Occupational Therapy, 49,* 695–702.

VanLeit, B. (1995). Using the case method to develop clinical reasoning skills in problem-based learning. *American Journal of Occupational Therapy, 49,* 349–353.

Wood, W. (1998). Nationally Speaking—The genius within. *American Journal of Occupational Therapy, 52,* 320–325.

Yerxa, E. J. (1995). Nationally Speaking—Who is the keeper of occupational therapy's practice and knowledge? *American Journal of Occupational Therapy, 49,* 295–299.

Yerxa, E. J. (1998a). Health and human spirit for occupation. *American Journal of Occupational Therapy, 52,* 412–422.

Yerxa, E. J. (1998b). Occupation: The keystone of a curriculum for a self-defined profession. *American Journal of Occupational Therapy, 52,* 365–372.

ACADEMIC LEADERSHIP

Introducing an Awareness of Cultural Diversity Into an Established Curriculum

Diana M. Bailey

Diana M. Bailey, EdD, OTR, FAOTA, is an Associate Professor, Tufts University, Boston School of Occupational Therapy, Medford, Massachusetts. This article resulted from a presentation at the 12th International Congress of the World Federation of Occupational Therapists, Montreal, Quebec, Canada, May 31 to June 5, 1998.

This article describes a diversity awareness program that was introduced into an established occupational therapy curriculum to increase students' awareness and appreciation of cultural diversity. An overview of the literature describing other methods for diversity awareness in health care curricula follows the rationale for using an infusion model for the program. The infusion model in this particular occupational therapy program includes a mandatory orientation for incoming students, ongoing faculty training, a wide variety of client types throughout academic and practice experiences, and establishing a safe environment in the classroom.

In the United States and in many other parts of the world, occupational therapy practitioners are finding that their work brings them into contact with clients from increasingly diverse backgrounds. In concert with the idea of a "global village," we find ourselves interacting with clients and coworkers from cultures other than our own. Our students must be prepared, knowledgeable, and sensitive to clients' deeply held, culturally bound, and idiosyncratic values and beliefs.

At the same time, we are finding that many of these students, who are themselves from diverse backgrounds, are experiencing nonacceptance and harassment in our colleges (Bodinger-deUriarte, 1991; Chacon, 1998a; Loo & Rolison, 1986; Steele, 1992). Thus, higher education facilities are appropriate places to begin addressing this lack of cultural sensitivity and acceptance. One approach is to broaden academic diversity in the teaching ranks, in the student body, and in curriculum content. Recent newspaper accounts have described research projects in Massachusetts that examined whether a diverse student body improves the quality of education (Chacon, 1998b) and who benefits and who loses from faculty and student discussions in the academy about increased diversity ("The Campus Move to Diversity," 1998). The third article (Chacon, 1998a) described the hostile atmosphere that gay and lesbian students experience on some college campuses.

About 3 years ago, faculty members of the Boston School of Occupational Therapy (BSOT) decided to add a new focus to our long-established program. We decided to introduce an awareness and an appreciation of cultural diversity. We wanted to do this for several reasons:

- so that students would be sensitive to differences among their clients and coworkers,
- so that students could work with clients to design culturally appropriate treatment plans, and
- so that students could more realistically help clients prepare to return to their own cultural, family, and community environments.

An additional benefit we hope to achieve is that students will be more interested and excited to learn about cultural differences among their fellow students, which will lead to a more open and accepting atmosphere in the university. As the popular media and personal experiences have shown us, and although we do not like to admit it, some college students still fear and have animosity toward persons of different cultures. Our goal is to provide the best educational experience possible for all students.

An Infusion Model

We believed that the most effective way to bring about cultural awareness was to use an infusion model whereby we introduce the topic in a multifaceted fashion throughout the curriculum. This model is somewhat similar to the curriculum enhancement project of MacPhee, Kreutzer, and Fritz (1994) in which they infused multicultural content into a sequence of four human development courses. Benefits of the project included reductions in prejudicial and blaming attitudes toward minority groups, increased knowledge of variations in human development, and inculcation of critical thinking skills. The authors believed that these effects were attributable to the "infusion of diversity throughout a single course (as opposed to mere exposure to developmental information in a typical course), and across a sequence of courses" (p. 713). Findings from this study suggest that attitudinal shifts may occur by making small changes in attitudes toward specific groups or issues. A cumulative effect was apparent from course to course as students moved through the sequence. "Such results suggest that a freestanding 'diversity day' or a single multicultural course will be less effective at enhancing multicultural sensibility" (MacPhee et al., 1994, p. 713).

Cultural Competence

To be effective occupational therapy practitioners, besides meeting professionally established educational standards, students must understand

- what the client role involves for persons of different cultures,
- what taking on the caregiver role involves and how other cultures perceive the helper role,
- what types of health care and treatment clients from a particular culture understand and accept, and
- which health care providers are acceptable to clients from cultures other than the student's own.

What do we mean by *culture*? In its *Uniform Terminology* document, the American Occupational Therapy Association (AOTA, 1994) defined culture as encompassing "customs, beliefs, activity patterns, behavior standards and expectations" (p. 1054) of a particular group. *Cultural competence* is the ability to provide health care that reflects an understanding of and respect for another culture. Culturally sensitive persons show an awareness, knowledge, and understanding of another's culture that leads to the adaptation of treatment to meet client needs, whereas persons who are culturally unaware lack understanding or sensitivity to different cultural needs.

In this endeavor at BSOT, we want students to gain an appreciation of cultural diversity, and we use an extremely broad definition of that term. We are interested in embracing all kinds of differences such as race and ethnicity, socioeconomic class, sexual orientation, religion, age, physical appearance (e.g., weight, height, disfigurement), ability and disability, and cognitive differences.

Cultural Diversity Programs in Health Care Education

Few published curricular innovations have described efforts to increase health care students' understanding of culture as it pertains to their interactions with clients. Efforts that exist are primarily in the nursing literature and seem to follow one of three approaches:

1. A one-time project or workshop in which students acquire and share cultural information. Dowling and Coppens (1996) wrote about an experiential learning project integrated into a sophomore nursing course in which small groups of students developed multimedia displays for staff members and students. In self-evaluations, students reported greater awareness of, sensitivity to, curiosity about, and appreciation of culture and its relationship to health practices.

    Rooda and Gay (1993) described a 1-day cultural sensitivity workshop for hospital nursing directors after which they generated cultural awareness strategies for training their own staff members. Workshop participants commented positively about the experience and believed that they could use what they had learned with their staff; however, the authors gave no evidence regarding whether participants actually did so.

2. A one-time course about all aspects of culture. Clinton (1996) described a required introductory course for baccalaureate-level nursing students in which they acquire theoretical knowledge of the relationships between cultural phenomena and health. Although the course objectives for students were clear, the article did not indicate whether the course was evaluated or whether the students achieved objectives. Lockhart and Resick (1997) described an undergraduate elective in their nursing program to develop students' cultural awareness and cross-cultural sensitivity. Course evaluations and follow-up surveys 1 year after the course indicated that students remembered the emotional effect of the experiential exercises and mentioned the long-term influence of learning strategies on their ability to provide culturally sensitive nursing care.

3. Threading cultural content across courses and throughout the curriculum (an infusion model). Henkle and Kennerly (1990) designed an integrated curriculum for baccalaureate-level nursing students to heighten students' awareness about the beliefs and values of peers in their own geographical area. Although the authors discussed no formal evaluation process, they indicated that students developed a new perspective about the appropriateness of using some nursing interventions for certain cultural groups and that students grew in their willingness to accept home remedies, dietary habits, and music as important parts of clients' health-related cultural perspectives.

Occupational Therapy Literature Concerning Cultural Diversity

Although several researchers have called for increased cultural knowledge and sensitivity on the part of occupational therapy practitioners (Dyck, 1989, 1991; Kinébanian & Stomph, 1992; Krefting & Krefting, 1991; Levine, 1987; Pope-Davis, Prieto, Whitaker, & Pope-Davis, 1993; Scott, 1997; Skawski, 1987), and some have described culturally sensitive treatment programs in occupational therapy (Dillard et al., 1992; Jungerson, 1992; Kanemoto, 1987; Tebbutt & Wade, 1985; Wieringa & McColl, 1987), only two studies described a curriculum intervention for occupational therapy students. First, Sayles-Folks and People (1990) described activities integrated into their "Orientation to Occupational Therapy" course, including simulation games, role-playing, values clarification, and critical thinking exercises: "The activities are designed to encourage the students to share their cultural backgrounds and perspectives, but to also value different perspectives and diversity" (p. 4). Students kept a weekly journal to record and reflect on their feelings and thoughts about the activities. The authors did not indicate whether the course was successful in achieving the goal "to provide a framework for understanding and communicating with all consumers" (p. 4).

Second, Yuen and Yau (1999) used a one-time project. They described a cultural interview experience during the students' first year and its effect (measured by self-report) on the students' cultural awareness and sensitivity toward another ethnic group. As a course assignment, students interviewed someone who either originated from another country or had spent at least 10 years in a foreign country and used an interview guide to become familiar with the sociocultural aspects of health and illness in a different country. Later surveys showed that 70% of the students said that the interview had a positive effect on their awareness of another cultural group, and about 45% said that the interview had a positive effect on their sensitivity and attitude toward another culture.

Decision To Adopt an Infusion Model

We decided that "squeezing" another course into an already overcrowded curriculum was not realistic. In addition, experience and the literature (MacPhee et al., 1994) have indicated that attitude change and knowledge gain are more likely to occur when material is dispersed throughout a program with an infusion model. We decided to encourage an overall appreciation of the differences in all of us. During their 2 years at BSOT, we expose the students to ideas about difference and sameness so that they can move from a position of tolerance of persons who are different from themselves, to respect, to appreciation of those differences, to enjoyment, and eventually to celebrating the diversity of others. Along the way, we hope to encourage our students in their quest to become sensitive practitioners who will provide meaningful treatment.

In class, we discuss the fact that dominant groups enjoy privileges, often without consciously being aware of this advantage (McIntosh, 1989), and the privileged group tends to hold the power. We discuss patterns of power, what it means to come from a power position, whether as a white person in a predominantly white culture, a person without disability in a predominantly able-bodied society, or as a practitioner in a helping relationship where the helper has the power.

What Methods Are We Using To Transmit This Message to Our Students and Our Faculty Members?

In striving to use an infusion model, we have searched for opportunities to introduce the notion of cultural differences into the curriculum and to help students gain an appreciation of that diversity. We have included learning experiences at many points throughout the program from orientation to Level II fieldwork and in many facets of the program, such as lectures, case presentations, client interviews in the classroom, experiential labs, fieldwork seminars, and fieldwork sites. Opportunities for learning are included for students, faculty members, and staff members. Specific experiences include the following.

Mandatory Orientation

In September of 1997, 1998, and 1999, at the beginning of the school year, we organized a mandatory session for incoming students entitled, Considering Diversity in Preparation for Practice. The session occurs before the new students have attended any classes, thus affording them the opportunity to get to know one another at the beginning of their program. No faculty members were allowed at the 1997 session to avoid inhibiting students from participating fully in discussions and activities. However, in 1998 and 1999, we decided to include as many faculty members as wanted to attend to show students that we are all involved in this endeavor together and that learning about cultural issues is an ongoing process.

Led by a university diversity trainer, students engaged in activities that allowed them to

- become aware of and celebrate their own differences,
- examine their own stereotypes,
- examine their own internalized oppression,
- take pride in their own group,
- identify power groups, and
- examine the role of power in maintaining oppressed groups.

A month later, we used an anonymous written questionnaire to ask students for feedback about the session. Not unexpectedly, feedback ranged from those who found the session to be a great opportunity to examine their own thoughts and feelings about diversity to a few who were unable to engage in the process in any meaningful way for various personal reasons.

Some positive comments included, "I'm now thinking about power some more and identifying hidden differences among us that make us unique," and "It made me more aware of myself and how I interact with others based on how I perceive them." Some of the students who did not find the session helpful gave such feedback as, "I didn't learn anything new, but it was a good chance to meet people in the class and see our differences and similarities," and "This topic is best taught outside the classroom because we do not truly learn about other cultures by hearing about them in school."

As we were planning the diversity orientation for our incoming students in September 1999, we asked for input from the past two classes regarding what we should change and what should remain the same. They have been helpful in telling us which activities and content made a lasting impression on them and which activities they found too difficult or not helpful.

Faculty Training

Obviously, providing incoming students with a diversity workshop was not enough. Remember, we had decided to use an infusion model to distribute the material throughout the curriculum. Before we could do this, faculty members had to participate in some training themselves, and this has become an ongoing part of our jobs.

Faculty training involves the same skilled university trainer who led the student workshop and thus far has consisted of an introduction to the concepts of inculcating diversity into a curriculum (in which we learned through participating in active exercises) and ongoing meetings with the trainer to develop case examples for use in the classroom (and which we continue to develop and discuss). In the future, we plan to hold regular faculty meetings to discuss various diverse groups of clients with whom our students are likely to be working in their future practices, to help each other incorporate diverse case examples into our teaching, and to help each other develop strategies to respond to students' questions or comments regarding diversity. We must develop the ability to handle highly charged situations that may arise as a result of introducing such topics as stereotypes, oppression, prejudice, and power.

Including Diverse Clients in Teaching

The third way that we are attempting to infuse diversity material throughout the curriculum is by encouraging and assisting each other to add a wide variety of client types to our teaching in the following ways:

- By including case examples in lectures and labs. An example is a consultant report that students write to promote procedural clinical reasoning. Students receive a detailed case study, and before attempting to analyze the case, they assign a cultural or ethnic identity and group to the client and family member or significant other. Their analysis should reflect the cultural mores of the chosen group.

- By inviting diverse guest lecturers who are often clients or former clients. For example, in an interactive clinical reasoning seminar, three groups of guest speakers "tell their story" to small groups of students, followed by a group interview of the guest. Guests are persons who have experienced spinal cord injury, those who are living with persistent mental illness, and those with AIDS or HIV infection. These same guests come from diverse racial or ethnic backgrounds (e.g., Hispanic, Asian, Italian, and African-American clients) and may have physical conditions such as low vision, loss of a hand, diabetes, and hepatitis. Students should frame their interview questions in ways that focus on the guests' perspectives of their hopes and dreams and the realities of living with a disability within the context of their culture.

- By including cultural issues in required course readings. In a management course that includes a module on ethics, students read and comment on material describing discriminatory hiring practices for persons living with AIDS and persons with diverse religious beliefs and practices and the experiences of a black occupational therapy manager. The following are students' comments resulting from this experience.
    — "As I read this article, I stopped part-way through to double-check the date it was published. I could not believe the experiences this woman encountered really occurred in the health care field in this decade. I suppose my response is naive and typical of an educated nonminority."
    — "Last summer, on my Level II, I experienced firsthand some instances of racism. My supervisor was a Haitian woman, and often it was only the two of us in the clinic. [The student is a Caucasian woman.] Once a man

(white, middle-aged) came in and introduced himself as a lawyer, and without giving either of us a chance to speak, explained a situation his client was experiencing after an on-the-job injury and that he wanted to have her reevaluated. He directed his whole story to me, basically ignoring my supervisor."

- By using fieldwork placements with diverse groups of clients.
- By including field assignments where students observe, record, and interview a wide variety of people. For example, one of our clinical reasoning seminars requires students to study a diverse group and write a short ethnography describing that group.

Safety in the Classroom

A final point, and one of the first lessons that we learned as classroom teachers during this project, is that, when you introduce material that addresses a person's values and cultural norms, you open up yourself and the rest of the class to the potential for feelings of discomfort, to intensely emotional responses, and, hence, to highly charged situations. We learned that if we want students to examine their personally held values, then we must give them a safe environment in which to do so. For this reason, many faculty members set ground rules in their classes. These rules include asking that students

- be fully present and participatory in all sessions,
- listen attentively to one another,
- maintain the confidentiality of personal statements made in class, and
- speak only from their own personal experience rather than from what others have told them or from stereotypes.

Several faculty members have attended a 2-day workshop that the university diversity trainer offers on ways to handle highly charged classroom situations. This workshop is open to all members of the university, and sharing difficult situations and coping strategies with faculty members from other departments has been an invaluable experience.

How Will We Evaluate the Effectiveness of the Model?

We are still evaluating and modifying our infusion method for threading an appreciation of diversity throughout the curriculum. Currently, we are examining several tools to find a standardized instrument, but as yet, we have not found a satisfactory way to evaluate the success of the program in terms of our objective (to raise students' cultural awareness and sensitivity). We will likely use attitude measures such as McConahay's (1986) Modern Racism Scale and Old Fashioned Racism Scale and MacDonald's (1972) Poverty Scale. Because we have been unable to find a standardized instrument to measure knowledge gains in complex multicultural issues, we will probably use qualitative methods to uncover themes of meaning related to diversity across program content and across the student body. At several points throughout the curriculum, we will continue to use self-evaluation and self-reflection logs regarding any awareness or attitude change that students believe they have achieved.

Summary

We expect to keep modifying all of our activities in an attempt to attain a fully multicultural and diverse occupational therapy program, one that allows all of us to celebrate human differences. Our ultimate aim is for our students to achieve the goals spelled out in the *Guidelines to the Occupational Therapy Code of Ethics*:

> to develop an understanding and appreciation for different cultures in order to provide culturally competent service. Culturally competent practitioners are aware of how service delivery can be affected by economic, ethnic, racial, geographic, gender, religious, and political factors as well as marital status, sexual orientation, and disability. (AOTA, 1998, p. 882) ▪

References

American Occupational Therapy Association. (1994). Uniform terminology for occupational therapy—Third edition. *American Journal of Occupational Therapy, 48*, 1047–1054.

American Occupational Therapy Association. (1998). Guidelines to the occupational therapy code of ethics. *American Journal of Occupational Therapy, 52,* 881–884.

Bodinger-deUriarte, C. (1991, December). The rise of hate crime on school campuses. *Phi Delta Kappa Research Bulletin,* 1–6.

The campus move to diversity: New viewpoints prompt new, layered ways of teaching. (1998, April 13). *The Boston Globe,* p. G3.

Chacon, R. (1998a, March 27). State program seeks to improve campus climate for gays and lesbians. *The Boston Globe,* p. 9.

Chacon, R. (1998b, April 17). Colleges try to prove diversity is valuable. *The Boston Globe,* pp. Al, A10.

Clinton, J. F. (1996). Cultural diversity and health care in America: Knowledge fundamental to cultural competence in baccalaureate nursing students. *Journal of Cultural Diversity, 3,* 4–8.

Dillard, M., Andonian, L., Flores, O., Lai, L., MacRae, A., & Shakir, M. (1992). Culturally competent occupational therapy in a diversely populated mental health setting. *American Journal of Occupational Therapy, 46,* 721–726.

Dowling, J., & Coppens, N. (1996). Understanding culture and health practices through an experiential learning project. *Nurse Educator, 21,* 43–46.

Dyck, I. (1989). The immigrant client: Issues in developing culturally sensitive practice. *Canadian Journal of Occupational Therapy, 56,* 248–255.

Dyck, I. (1991). Multiculturalism and occupational therapy: Sharing the challenge. *Canadian Journal of Occupational Therapy, 58,* 224–226.

Henkle, J., & Kennerly, S. (1990). Cultural diversity: A resource in planning and implementing nursing care. *Public Health Nursing, 7,* 145–149.

Jungerson, K. (1992). Culture, theory, and the practice of occupational therapy in New Zealand/Aotearoa. *American Journal of Occupational Therapy, 46,* 745–750.

Kanemoto, J. S. (1987). Cultural implications in treatment of Japanese-American patients. *Occupational Therapy in Health Care, 4,* 115–125.

Kinébanian, A., & Stomph, M. (1992). Cross-cultural occupational therapy: A critical reflection. *American Journal of Occupational Therapy, 46,* 751–757.

Krefting, L., & Krefting, D. (1991). Cultural influences on performance. In C. Christiansen & C. Baum (Eds.), *Occupational therapy: Overcoming human performance deficits* (pp. 100–122). Thorofare, NJ: Slack.

Levine, R. (1987). Culture: A factor influencing the outcomes of occupational therapy. *Occupational Therapy in Health Care, 4,* 3–16.

Lockhart, J., & Resick, L. (1997). Teaching cultural competence: The value of experiential learning and community resources. *Nurse Educator, 22,* 27–31.

Loo, C., & Rolison, G. (1986). Alienation of ethnic minority students at a predominantly white university. *Journal of Higher Education, 57,* 58–77.

MacDonald, A., Jr. (1972). More on the Protestant ethic. *Journal of Consulting and Clinical Psychology, 39,* 116–122.

MacPhee, D., Kreutzer, J., & Fritz, J. (1994). Infusing a diversity perspective into human development courses. *Child Development, 65,* 699–715.

McConahay, J. (1986). Modern racism, ambivalence, and the Modern Racism Scale. In J. Dovidio & S. Gaertner (Eds.), *Prejudice, discrimination, and racism.* Orlando, FL: Academic.

McIntosh, P. (1989, July/August). White privilege: Unpacking the invisible knapsack. *Peace and Freedom,* 10–12.

Pope-Davis, D. B., Prieto, L.R., Whitaker, C.M., & Pope-Davis, S. A. (1993). Exploring multicultural competencies of occupational therapists: Implications for education and training. *American Journal of Occupational Therapy, 47,* 838–844.

Rooda, L., & Gay, G. (1993). Staff development for culturally sensitive nursing care. *Journal of Nursing Staff Development, 9,* 262–265.

Sayles-Folks, S., & People, L. (1990, September). Cultural sensitivity training for occupational therapists. *Physical Disabilities Special Interest Section Newsletter, 13,* 4–5.

Scott, R. (1997). Investigation of cross-cultural practice: Implications for curriculum development. *Canadian Journal of Occupational Therapy, 64,* 89–96.

Skawski, K. A. (1987). Ethnic/racial considerations in occupational therapy: A survey of attitudes. *Occupational Therapy in Health Care, 4,* 37–47.

Steele, C. (1992). Race and the schooling of black Americans. *Atlantic, 269,* 68–78.

Tebbutt, M., & Wade, B. (1985). Frames of reference in the care of migrant patients. *Australian Journal of Occupational Therapy, 32,* 91–103.

Wieringa, N., & McColl, M. (1987). Implications of the Model of Human Occupation for intervention with native Indians. *Occupational Therapy in Health Care, 4,* 73–91.

Yuen, H., & Yau, M. (1999). Cross-cultural awareness and occupational therapy education. *Occupational Therapy International, 6*(1), 24–34.

Suggested Readings

Bagasao, P. (1989, November/December). Student voices: Breaking the silence: The Asian and Pacific American experience. *Change,* 28–37.

Fuss, D. (1990). Essentialism in the classroom. In D. Fuss (Ed.), *Essentially speaking* (pp. 113–119). New York: Routledge Kegan & Paul.

Gerschick, T. (1993). Should and can a white, heterosexual, middle-class man teach students about social inequality and oppression? One person's experience and reflections. In D. Shoem, M. Frankel, S. Zuniga, & S. Lewis (Eds.), *Multicultural teaching in the university* (pp. 200–207). Westport, CT: Greenwood.

Hoy, R. (1993). Clashing cultures: A "model minority" speaks out on cultural shyness. *Science, 262,* 1117–1118.

Puccio, P. (1991). Teachers' lives, students' lives: Some reflections. In J. Nyquist, R. Abbott, D. Wulff, & J. Sprague (Eds.), *Preparing the professorate of tomorrow to teach: Selected Readings in TA training* (pp. 105–109). Dubuque, IA: Kendall/Hunt.

Sleeter, C. (1993). How white teachers construct race. In D. Shoem, M. Frankel, S. Zuniga, & S. Lewis (Eds.), *Multicultural teaching in the university* (pp. 157–171). Westport, CT: Greenwood.

Smith, D. (1991). The challenge of diversity: Alienation in the academy and its implications for faculty. *Journal on Excellence in College Teaching, 2,* 129–137.

Tatum, B. D. (1992). Talking about race, learning about racism: The application of racial identity development theory in the classroom. *Harvard Educational Review, 62*(1), 1–24.

Resource

National Coalition Building Institute International (NCBI)
1835 K Street, NW
Suite 715
Washington, DC 20006

The NCBI is a nonprofit leadership training organization established in 1984 to eliminate prejudice and intergroup conflicts in communities throughout the world. Chapters exist in Canada, England, Switzerland, and the United States.

ACADEMIC LEADERSHIP

Brief Processes for Admission to Occupational Therapy Programs: A Performance-Based Model

Lillian Kaplan

Lillian Kaplan, MA, OTR, BCP, is Acting Program Director and Assistant Professor, York College, City University of New York, Department of Health Sciences, Jamaica, New York.

Despite a current increase in the quality and quantity of applicants to occupational therapy programs, a lack of diversity remains in the student population. The profession has made efforts to attract minority candidates; however, this goal has remained separate from the discussion of admission objectives. The increase in students has caused many faculty members to review criteria and revise screening methods. These revisions have the potential to define the future makeup of the profession. This article presents a performance-based model that involves the tenet of using activity to elicit integrated behavior. This model involves a practical examination that uses craft activities to measure collaborative behaviors. We offer this model as an alternative admissions method that is inclusive of a diverse student population.

Occupational therapy is experiencing an increase in the amount of available educational programs as well as in the quality and quantity of applicants. Although the profession is expanding, it is maintaining a lack of diversity (Stancliff, 1997). This dilemma requires that educators begin to examine admissions procedures for occupational therapy programs. Faculty reviews and revisions of admission criteria can change methods of student selection and thereby have the potential to define the makeup of the profession for years to come. The purpose of this article is to offer a model for admissions to occupational therapy programs that includes a performance-based practical examination.

A general consensus exists regarding the type of student that occupational therapy programs seek (i.e., students with diverse cultures, genders, socioeconomic backgrounds, and internal motivations; self-knowledge; good academic skills). However, a general dissatisfaction is evident regarding the current methods for measuring these personal and qualitative characteristics (Heater, 1995; McEwen & Crawford, 1995).

Faculty time constraints, the quest for efficiency, and the emphasis on objectivity in decision making have shifted the focus of many programs' admissions criteria toward objective measures. These measures include standardized test scores, the type of institution previously attended, specific course grades, and grade point average (GPA). The admissions process of York College in Jamaica, New York, has multiple criteria, one of which is a craft-based practical examination. This performance-based method quantifies learning and collaborative processes. Despite the wide use of these objective measures, little research has examined the implications of this admissions process for occupational therapy. Guinier (1997) found the emphasis on academic standing to heavily influence the demographics and characteristics of students admitted into professional studies. Reliance on the academic standard favors those applicants who are from higher socioeconomic backgrounds, attended private 4-year colleges, and are not distracted by financial and family responsibilities. GPA appears to be predictive only of some criteria of academic performance, such as exit GPA and completion of the academic program (Schmalz, Rahr, & Allen, 1990; Vargo, Madill, & Davidson, 1986). Standardized tests, such as the Scholastic Achievement Tests, the Survey of Interpersonal Values, or the Otis Quick Scoring Mental Ability Test, have been predictive only of those students who would drop out or withdraw from the academic program (Blaisdell & Gordon, 1979; Schmalz et al., 1990). Thus, measures of academic standing appear to be generally predictive of students' abilities to complete academic requirements, such as occupational therapy course work and certification examinations (Blaisdell & Gordon, 1979; Templeton, Burcham, & Franck, 1994; Vargo et al., 1986), but have not been shown to measure creativity and interpersonal skills, fieldwork success, or clinical performance with clients (Best, 1994; Kirchner & Holm, 1997; McEwen & Crawford, 1995).

Admissions criteria may also include subjective measures, such as interviews or writing samples. These items presumably measure characteristics that are essential to clinical success. Subjective methods appear to be rarely used in the absence of objective measures, so their specific predictive ability is unclear. Interviews are generally criticized for their subjectivity and time consumption. Applicants may rehearse questions, give pat answers, or demonstrate desired social skills, which undermines the process (Heater, 1995; McEwen & Crawford, 1995). The use of groups or specific behavioral criteria appears to influence the scoring of individual interviewers. These scoring differences can be decisive in the admission of a particular student (Mann, 1979; Shepard, 1980). However, the interview can indicate a student's clinical success because interviews can bring out the character traits of applicants, specifically their ability to form rapport when in a high-pressure or professional atmosphere (Foss, 1995; Shepard, 1980).

Submitted writing samples are likewise subjective and often reflect a student's use of multiple resources; thus, they are unreliable measures of academic or writing ability. In addition, information requested is often duplicated during the interview process. However, writing samples, either spontaneous or prepared, may be examples of an applicant's technical ability and critical thinking (Heater, 1995; McEwen & Crawford, 1995).

Programs often mix objective and subjective methods to obtain a more complete measure of an applicant's performance. Lucci and Brockway (1980), in a longitudinal study, demonstrated that objective and subjective measures used concurrently in the screening process predicted positive outcomes in both academic and clinical performance. However, Johnson, Arbes, and Thompson

(1974) showed that combinations of admission methods were not predictive of performance of different classes of students (e.g., students from different socioeconomic groups, transfer students from 4-year colleges vs. community colleges, minority students vs. white students, men vs. women). Embattled educators seeking efficiency and cost cutting have attempted to identify which method will adequately predict both academic and clinical success. Avi-Itzhak and Kellner (1992) and Bridle (1987) admitted students on the basis of objective or subjective methods in an attempt to identify which single admission measure predicted both academic and clinical performance. Both studies concluded that objective measures predicted academic and fieldwork performance and thus were more efficient methods of admission selection. Subjective measures were discontinued at their institutions. However, in both of these studies, students admitted solely because of subjective measures did equally well clinically, which may mean that both groups have equal potential to become good therapists. However, these programs now exclude students with less-than-stellar academic standing (for whatever reason). Thus, we must begin to examine the characteristics of groups that would be excluded when shifting admissions processes to forms of objective measures. Unfortunately, both of these studies did not report the relationship of socioeconomic status to prior educational experience and academic standing. These programs did not report on the diversity of their student populations or state that diversity was part of their admissions objectives.

Alternative models of student selection that diversify occupational therapy programs in culture, ethnicity, and life experience appear to be necessary. Fewer than 8% of occupational therapists practicing in the United States identify themselves as a member of a minority group, and similar underrepresentation is evident internationally (Rowe & MacDonald, 1995). The American Occupational Therapy Association (AOTA) is making an effort to recruit and retain persons from culturally diverse populations (Wells & Whiting, 1998); however, we cannot separate recruitment from the student selection processes in this effort. Motivated persons who do not meet objective screening criteria for professional programs may be turning to occupational therapy assistant programs, which have less stringent GPA standards (Wyrick & Stern, 1987). The AOTA Education Data Survey of 1995 (Rowe & MacDonald, 1995) showed that the percentages of minority students were consistently higher in occupational therapy assistant programs from 1987 through 1994, with significant differences of up to 9.6% between the two program levels. The use of heavily weighted GPA admission criteria in professional occupational therapy programs may discourage nontraditional mature students, students with backgrounds in crafts and media, and students with multiple role responsibilities (Heater, 1995; Simpson, 1997). Students in these groups may comprise the diverse student population we seek.

The York College Model

The occupational therapy program at York College seeks to include, via the admissions process, those persons with moderate academic standing and who have families, jobs, or other responsibilities that may preclude them from achieving high academic success. This process allows the York College occupational therapy professional program to select from a pool of candidates diverse in culture, maturity, and socioeconomic levels. The unique feature of York College's screening process is its inclusion of a heavily weighted performance-based practical examination. The practical examination involves the occupational therapy tenet that demonstration of competence is best observed from engagement in activity. In an academic context, this requires observation of students engaged in the process of learning, collaboration, and workmanship.

Despite the economic pressures and time constraints in clinical practice, York College occupational therapy faculty members maintain that a primary tenet of occupational therapy is collaboration between clinician and client. This ability comes from a person's experiences, culture, maturity, and coping and learning strategies that develop throughout the life span primarily outside academia. In many cultures, adult social competence occurs through interactive learning, task performance, and verbal reasoning. Development of competence outside of Western, middle-class contexts often involves demonstration, mentoring, imitation, and motor learning (Kagitcibasi, 1996). Therefore, the practical component of the admissions process examines those learning and collaborative behaviors that students bring to the profession.

The practical examination involves using crafts to elicit these complex behaviors. Occupational therapy practitioners have typically used crafts and activities to elicit, evaluate, and facilitate higher functioning behavior, and this concept is part of occupational therapy education (Allen & Allen, 1987; Breines, 1989). The use of a functional, goal-directed, and meaningful activity to evaluate a person's skills is inherently an occupational therapy method (Cymkin & Robinson, 1990; Fidler, 1981). In observing the performance of the craft, one has a window into the person's sensory, motor, cognitive, social, and psychological systems. In addition to observing a student learning, the practical examination elicits skills that demonstrate the student's ability to perform three types of collaborative processes.

1. Working jointly (working with or together with)
2. Assisting (which constitutes a learner and teacher relationship)
3. Cooperating (giving up one's needs for the larger good)

A student's GPA and academic course work, although important indicators of learned knowledge and academic ability, are not predictive criteria for skill in collaboration.

The Practical Examination Process at York College

Students receive hourly appointments for the day of the practical examination in groups of 12. On arrival, each student receives a number from 1 to 12. These numbers are the means of scoring individuals in that group. The students divide into groups of odd and even numbers. A faculty member leads each smaller group into separate classrooms that have stations for learning a craft (Figure 1). The odd-numbered group learns an origami task, and the even-numbered group learns a rubber stamping task. Students receive written instructions in step sequence for the task. The leader offers a model of each step for the origami task. All students have 5 min to learn and complete the task. Students receive (and are offered) no assistance. The learning segments of the practical examination are important for observations of students' abilities to follow written, verbal, or visual instruction under pressure independent of mistakes others are making. The students' work is collected for later scoring by the faculty members on the learning process, specifically step completion and workmanship. Both groups then come together in a third room with stations for the crafts just learned. Odd-numbered and even-numbered students pair up at these stations. In testing the collaborative ability of assisting, the odd-numbered students who just learned the origami task teach the even-numbered students who learned the rubber stamping craft.

Examiners consisting of York College occupational therapy faculty members move around the students and score teaching criteria (i.e., step explanation), teaching without doing for the learner, modification of instruction, rapport, and so forth. The even-numbered students then teach their rubber stamping craft, and examiners grade them on the same criteria.

The same partners stay together and go to new stations for a task requiring them to work jointly. Partners must produce one product from shared materials, written instructions, and a common model. This allows the evaluation of cooperation and ability to work jointly with a peer on the same goal. In this interaction, students must give up some of their own needs (to form a perfect product their way) to meet the needs of another and to be successful in the time allotted. Examiners grade students on such criteria as shared responsibilities for steps, give and take of ideas, sharing of materials, appropriateness of communications, and so forth. Next, odd-numbered students separate from even-numbered students at separate workstations. Each group learns a different embroidery stitch with written instructions, diagrams, and direct teaching assistance from the faculty members. After learning by doing a row of stitches, odd-numbered students pair with even-numbered students again. The examiners grade ability to assist as students teach their stitches to each other.

This sequence is repeated with each group of 12 until the examiners have evaluated all students. Each group practical examination takes 1 hr. Thus, we

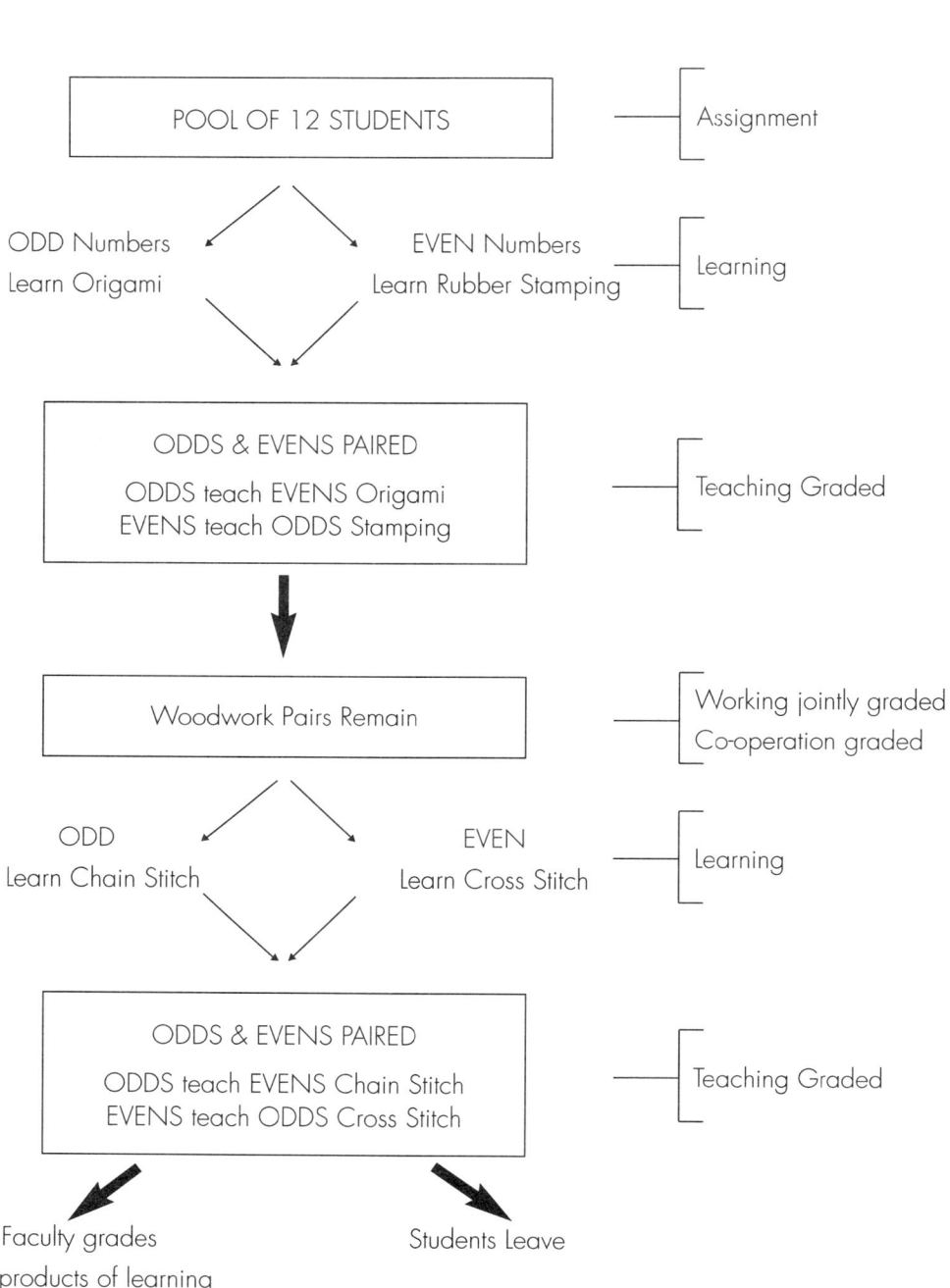

Figure 1. Practical examination flow chart depicts a sequential view of how students are separated and regrouped for observation of collaboration skills during the practical examination.

can evaluate up to 8 groups of 12 in 1 day. We chose the crafts so that some materials would be familiar and some unfamiliar across genders and cultures. We use the scores from the practical examination in conjunction with other measures, such as a required moderate GPA, letters of reference, an autobiographical sketch, and an interview by a small group consisting of occupational therapy clinical supervisors and faculty members. We weight all of these measures by percentile in accordance with faculty determination of the fundamental qualities of a successful student and clinician. We then rank the total scores for the screening process and select the top-ranked students. Students who fail the criteria of either the practical examination or the interview are excluded from the ranking process altogether.

Summary

The issue of admissions criteria for entry-level students is important in the light of its influence on the long-term composition of persons in the general profession. The professional occupational therapy program at York College is contributing to the diversification of the profession, is serving our immediate public community, and is following the mission of the college. Faculty members have used an inclusive process of selection rather than an exclusive one. York College's admissions process has multiple criteria, which include a craft-based practical examination. This performance-based method quantifies learning and collaborative processes. Further study is necessary to investigate the method's contribution to the 65% minority student population in York College's occupational therapy professional program (York College, 1998). This alternative admissions method allows York College's occupational therapy program to distinguish persons with moderate academic standing and financial and family responsibilities who have the potential to be excellent students and clinicians. Similarly, the practical examination may be a way of discriminating those persons with high GPAs who would be unsuccessful in fieldwork. A study is under way to examine the relationship of the practical evaluation to academic and clinical performance. ■

Acknowledgments

I thank Wimberly Edwards, MS, OTL, FAOTA, and Ruth Kreim, MA, OTR/L, for their foundational work on the practical examination and their assistance and collaboration. I also thank Rita Cottrell, MA, OTL, for her assistance in manuscript preparation.

References

Allen, C. K., & Allen, R. E. (1987). Cognitive disabilities: Measuring the social consequences of mental disorders. *Journal of Clinical Psychology, 48*(5), 185–190.

Avi-Itzhak, T., & Kellner, H. (1992). A longitudinal study for predicting performance in an occupational therapy program. *Israel Journal of Occupational Therapy, 1,* E11–E24.

Best, C. E. (1994). A prediction model of performance in Level II fieldwork in physical disabilities. *American Journal of Occupational Therapy, 48,* 926–931.

Blaisdell, E. A., Jr., & Gordon, D. (1979). Selection of occupational therapy students. *American Journal of Occupational Therapy, 33,* 223–229.

Breines, E. B. (1989). Media education based on the philosophy of pragmatism. *American Journal of Occupational Therapy, 43,* 461–464.

Bridle, M. (1987). Student selection: A comparison of three methods. *Canadian Journal of Occupational Therapy, 54,* 113–117.

Cymkin, S., & Robinson, A. (1990). *Occupational therapy and activities health: Toward health through activities.* Boston: Little, Brown.

Fidler, G. S. (1981). From crafts to competence. *American Journal of Occupational Therapy, 35,* 567–573.

Foss, J. J. (1995, June). Admissions dilemma. *Education Special Interest Section Newsletter, 5,* 2–3.

Guinier, L. (1997, June 24). The real bias in higher education. *The New York Times,* p. A19:2.

Heater, S. L. (1995, March). On student admissions: Confessions of an academically challenged professor. *Education Special Interest Section Newsletter, 5,* 2–4.

Johnson, R. W., Arbes, B. H., & Thompson, C. G. (1974). Selection of occupational therapy students. *American Journal of Occupational Therapy, 28,* 597–601.

Kagitcibasi, C. (1996). *Family and human development across cultures: A view from the other side.* Mahwah, NJ: Erlbaum.

Kirchner, G. L, & Holm, M. B. (1997). Prediction of academic and clinical performance of occupational therapy students in an entry-level master's program. *American Journal of Occupational Therapy, 51,* 775–779.

Lucci, J. A., & Brockway, J. A. (1980). Student selection process: A follow-up study. *American Journal of Occupational Therapy, 34,* 27–32.

Mann, W. C. (1979). Interview scoring differences in student selection interviews. *American Journal of Occupational Therapy, 33,* 235–239.

McEwen, M., & Crawford, L. K. (1995, March). The admissions process: In search of congruity in practice. *Education Special Interest Section Newsletter, 5,* 1–2.

Rowe, N., & MacDonald, R. (1995). Minority ethnic groups and occupational therapy: Part I: Recruitment of students. *British Journal of Occupational Therapy, 58,* 256–260.

Schmalz, G., Rahr, R., & Allen, R. (1990). The use of pre-admission data to predict levels of success in allied health students. *Occupational Therapy Journal of Research, 10,* 367–377.

Shepard, K. (1980). Use of small group interviews for selection into allied health educational programs. *Journal of Allied Health, 9*(2), 85–94.

Simpson, K. (1997). Editorial: Are we picking from the wrong barrel? *Advance for Occupational Therapists, 13*(42), 3.

Stancliff, B. (1997). Recruiting ethnic students calls for innovation. *OT Practice, 2,* 13–14.

Templeton, M., Burcham, A., & Franck, L. (1994). Predictive study of physical therapy admission variables. *Journal of Allied Health, 23*(2), 79–87.

Vargo, J., Madill, H., & Davidson, P. (1986). The pre-admission interview as a predictor of academic grades and fieldwork performance. *Canadian Journal of Occupational Therapy, 53,* 211–215.

Wells, S., & Whiting, F. (1998). A celebration of diversity: Reviewing AOTA's progress toward creating a more diverse profession. *OT Practice, 3,* 31–34.

Wyrick, J. M., & Stern, E. B. (1987). The recruitment of occupational therapy students: A national survey. *American Journal of Occupational Therapy, 41,* 173–178.

York College. (1998). [Occupational therapy program database of student profiles from 1994–1998]. Unpublished raw data.

INVITED ARTICLES

Expanding the Utility of Scholarly Activity: Three Views

Our aim in this discussion is to share several strategies for linking scholarly activity to other functions in occupational therapy practice. We shall establish three useful links for scholarship: continued education, clinical and management functions, and graduate education. Our collective aim is to share strategies for linking various functions in practice that are often separated.

This article was nested within a mini course at the 1999 American Occupational Therapy Association (AOTA) Annual Conference and Exposition in Indianapolis, Indiana. Patricia Crist, Editor of Innovations in Occupational Therapy Education, *asked us to see the potential for this piece within our presentation. The kind of nesting that this article represents (that of casting an oral presentation into a written format) is familiar to many. Herein, we discuss a less familiar form of nesting—that of linking scholarly activity to continued education, clinical and management functions, and graduate education. We share strategies that have worked for us. We tell personal stories (rarely told) about the goodness of fit and strength of these links. We hope to expand, in a practical way, the utility of scholarly activity.*

Two key terms appear throughout this discussion, and they warrant defining. We accept the meaning of the term utility *that we find in most dictionaries: usefulness, the power to satisfy needs or wants, practical usage. We note a rather circular definition of* scholarly activity *in dictionaries (any activity associated with the methods of scholars), and so we use Mosey's (1998) definition instead: "Intellectual activities identified by the scholarly community as being most likely to culminate in the creation of sound, abstract information....A scholar may be a historian, theologian, scientist, or philosopher" (p. 761).*

Our titles use a metaphor, the making of links. This metaphor is kin to those of nesting, orchestrating, or folding. All of these imply some relatedness, fit, or congruence among concepts that beg connecting. To see the shape of a link is to see the actions of arms and hands as they nest one object within another, to fold items together, or to orchestrate a union of voices.

Picture a set of nesting eggs, four of them in a row. If the largest nesting egg that you see represents a scholarly presentation at the state level, you may see within it some potential for a presentation at a national conference. That becomes the second egg. And within that egg may nest potential for a peer-reviewed article (the third egg). Within the article may nest a book chapter (the last egg). Within that first presentation nested the prospect of others. The question one asks with nesting is, "What other activity might link with this one?" We contrast this metaphor with another com-

monly used—*juggling. Juggling is a breathtaking and deft handling of items. Nesting, or making links, seems more efficient and less stressful than the act of tossing objects into the air and hoping to catch them. We hope that the strategies in this discussion emerge as efficient and helpful mechanisms that practitioners can master and teach to students.*

—Suzanne M. Peloquin, PhD, OTR, FAOTA

Reference

Mosey, A. C. (1998). The competent scholar. *American Journal of Occupational Therapy, 52,* 760–764.

INVITED ARTICLES

Establishing Links With Continued Education

Suzanne M. Peloquin

Suzanne M. Peloquin, PhD, OTR, FAOTA, is Professor, Department of Occupational Therapy, School of Allied Health Sciences, the University of Texas Medical Branch at Galveston, Galveston, Texas.

This discussion shows the manner in which one educator uses scholarly works either to create or to enhance varied learning opportunities relating to practice: presentations at local, state, and national levels; workshops and in-service presentations; articles in practice magazines and newsletters; computer-based information services; correspondence courses (either text-based or technological); and texts and monographs that practitioners use.

I shall link two professional functions: scholarly activity, as defined in the introduction, and continued education. I understand *continued education* to mean the varied learning opportunities associated with formal education and related to practice. When I think of continuing education, I think of the following: presentations at local, state, and national levels; workshops and in-service presentations; articles in practice magazines and newsletters; computer-based information services; correspondence courses (either text-based or technological); and texts and monographs that practitioners use. Because many of these same opportunities occur in formal educational programs that emphasize practice, I will discuss the links possible in undergraduate education as I discuss continued education.

To illustrate this linking mode, I will share the manner in which I have nested my scholarly work into continued education activities by using articles published in *The American Journal of Occupational Therapy* (*AJOT*) during the past several years (Peloquin, 1988, 1989a, 1989b, 1990, 1991a, 1991b, 1993a, 1993b, 1994, 1995a, 1995b, 1996a, 1996b, 1996c). My decision to use this work is deliberate. When persons comment on my scholarly activity, they use these descriptors: anecdotal, artful, phenomenological, esoteric, literary, philosophical, historical, theoretical, and conceptual. Such work seems so far "off the beaten path" that on a continuum of utility, it seems marginal. My work thus seems apt to consider. If esoteric work might become continued education, how much more so might traditional scholarship?

Linking for the Sake of Relevance

One overarching strategy has led to my forging links with practical venues such as presentations and workshops, faculty and curricular development functions, and pieces within practice and educational literature. That strategy has been the coupling of my esoteric work with that perceived to be more relevant. Consider, for example, a cluster of *AJOT* articles that together explore the art of practice. These articles fall into a philosophical group, which is evident in their titles: "The Depersonalization of Patients" (Peloquin, 1993b), "Sustaining the Art of Practice" (Peloquin, 1989b), "The Patient–Therapist Relationship in Occupational Therapy" (Peloquin, 1990), and "Beliefs That Shape Care" (Peloquin, 1993a). Another grouping has an artful (and thus less useful) theme: "The Fullness of Empathy" (Peloquin, 1995b), "Art: An Occupation With Promise for Developing Empathy" (Peloquin, 1996a), and "Occupational Therapy as Art and Science" (Peloquin, 1994). This work on the art of practice invited coupling with something else.

By linking this cluster of articles to work from the social sciences and by seeking help from a colleague and coauthor, Debora Davidson, MS, OTR, on some projects, I have blended work on the art of practice into continuing education. Salient information on more "usable" constructs such as verbal and nonverbal communication, learning and teaching styles, or active listening has moved esoteric material to the useful end of the continuum. A listing of these activities may become suggestions for others: Create an elective undergraduate course on interpersonal skills; present this course as a workshop at state and national levels; publish a "Brief or New" (practice-related) piece in *AJOT* (Peloquin & Davidson, 1993); create, with savvy practitioners (e.g., Laurita Fike, MA, OTR, then at Texas Woman's University), weekend workshops for clinicians; offer the original course at another university; synthesize educational constructs and offer this "chunk" as faculty or curricular development workshops (five to date); write a "Brief or New" piece about using the arts (Peloquin, 1996c); and craft a set of teaching manuals for either the classroom or the clinic (Davidson & Peloquin, 1998). The overarching strategy (coupling for the sake of relevance to practice) is one that works.

Making Cameos

Another strategy, less overarching but helpful, merits mention: "bite-sizing" or "cameo-making," in which the useful act is that of making large scholarly works more practical by using imaging or metaphors that help others to see connections. A second grouping of my articles shows how bite-sizing or cameo-making can serve continuing education. These are historical articles such as "Occupational Therapy Service: Individual and Collective Understandings of the Founders" (Peloquin, 1991a, 1991b) and "Moral Treatment" (Peloquin, 1989a, 1994). An adage from high school, "Why we study history is always such a mystery," sums the views of many. The linking strategy for this historical work was to carve small parts (less than 125 words) from these articles and note their lasting relevance. The end result was this: 24 of these cameos appeared for 2 years in *Revista OT*, the newsletter of the Texas Occupational Therapy Association (TOTA), in a column called "Keepsakes." The monthly byline near the title changed the old adage: "Occupational therapy history remains a source of continued learning. 'Keepsakes' aims to use that source and generate reflection."

The idea of bite-sizing or cameo-making found another home. As I met in a planning session with editors Maureen Neistadt, ScD, OTR/L, FAOTA, and Betty Crepeau, PhD, OTR, FAOTA, for the ninth edition of *Willard and Spackman's Occupational Therapy* (1998), I shared my regret that history was often in a separate chapter and at risk for disregard. I wondered aloud if practice chapters might be linked with historical themes. The result of that discussion was the creation of 49 "recurring displays" or boxes in the textbook (12 of them historical) that we honed from the "Keepsakes" columns. The 37 other displays linked research and ethical themes (likewise often less valued) to practice chapters.

Linking for the Sake of Understanding

The last strategy that I shall mention is another "coupling for the sake of relevance" but with a twist. This link appears in "Doubletakes," a column in its fourth year in *Revista OT*. The column aims to promote research among those who find it daunting. The idea emerged during a discussion within a newly established TOTA Research Committee that I had been asked to join. Given my skewed scholarly bent, I saw a coupling that might let my use of metaphor work to some advantage.

The coupling was this: Two persons would write a column, one to explain research elements (less than 200 words) and the other (me) to take a common sense view of these elements (from 45 to 75 words). Each writer would have a distinct "take" on research, hence the title. Patterned after the news column "Click and Clack," in which brothers solve car woes, "Doubletakes" has had two research contributors: Margarette Shelton, MS, OTR, then a doctoral student a Texas Woman's University and a clinician at the University of Texas Medical Branch Galveston Hospitals, wrote during the first year, and Beatriz Abreu, PhD, OTR, FAOTA, a local colleague, researcher, and coauthor, followed.

The column's work, as both Shelton and Abreu explained (independently of each other) was to "demystify" research. In one column, Shelton explained experimental design. My "take" on her explanation was as follows:

> Within this research design, analysis seems to be a matter of comparing. It seems a much more rigorous but still familiar version of actions we take on the day-to-day. For example, when I make a couple of batches of cookies and run out of chocolate chips for the second batch, I might compare the two along the dimension of taste or chocolate flavor and find one lacking. (Peloquin & Shelton, 1997, p. 6)

A year later, Abreu discussed research as a tool for both basic and applied inquiry. My take was as follows:

> This discussion about research as a tool makes me think of another—a claw hammer. The claw hammer is a single tool that can function in more than one way. I can use the hammer to seal something securely in place (applied inquiry),

or I can use the claw end to open up a brand new container (basic inquiry). (Abreu & Peloquin, 1998, p. 7)

In this fourth year of the column, Abreu and I are making cameos from our *AJOT* article "Competence in Scientific Inquiry and Research" (Abreu, Peloquin, & Ottenbacher, 1998). The coupling in "Doubletakes" adds this twist: Metaphor (a strategy drawn from the arts) makes research more practical. The byline for this column reads: "Research—the term invites repeated searches into its meaning."

The linking mode for expanding the utility of scholarly activity within this first brief article is that of seeing nested within scholarly articles the potential for continued education opportunities and then acting on that potential. The kind of work that expands the utility of scholarship also enhances a person's connections with others. The theme of collaborating with others, an act so far-reaching and rewarding, thus recurs throughout our three discussions of scholars who connect with educators, managers, and practitioners. ∎

References

Abreu, B. A., & Peloquin, S. M. (1998). Doubletakes. *Revista OT, 63,* 7.

Abreu, B., Peloquin, S. M., & Ottenbacher, K. (1998). Competence in scientific inquiry and research. *American Journal of Occupational Therapy, 52,* 751–759.

Davidson, D. A., & Peloquin, S. M. (1998). *Making connections with others: A handbook on interpersonal practice.* Bethesda, MD: American Occupational Therapy Association.

Neistadt, M. E., & Crepeau, E. B. (Eds.). (1998). *Willard and Spackman's occupational therapy* (9th ed.). Philadelphia: Lippincott.

Peloquin, S. M. (1988). Linking purpose to procedure during interactions with patients. *American Journal of Occupational Therapy, 42,* 775–781.

Peloquin, S. M. (1989a). Looking Back—Moral treatment: Contexts considered. *American Journal of Occupational Therapy, 43,* 537–544.

Peloquin, S. M. (1989b). Sustaining the art of practice in occupational therapy. *American Journal of Occupational Therapy, 43,* 219–226.

Peloquin, S. M. (1990). The patient–therapist relationship in occupational therapy: Understanding visions and images. *American Journal of Occupational Therapy, 44,* 13–21.

Peloquin, S. M. (1991a). Looking Back—Occupational therapy service: Individual and collective understandings of the founders, part 1. *American Journal of Occupational Therapy, 45,* 353–360.

Peloquin, S. M. (1991b). Looking Back—Occupational therapy service: Individual and collective understanding of the founders, part 2. *American Journal of Occupational Therapy, 45,* 733–744.

Peloquin, S. M. (1993a). Patient–therapist relationship: Beliefs that shape care. *American Journal of Occupational Therapy, 47,* 935–942.

Peloquin, S. M. (1993b). The depersonalization of patients: A profile gleaned from narratives. *American Journal of Occupational Therapy, 47,* 830–837.

Peloquin, S. M. (1994). The Issue Is—Occupational therapy as art and science: Should the older definition be reclaimed? *American Journal of Occupational Therapy, 48,* 1083–1096.

Peloquin, S. M. (1995a). The Issue Is—Communication skills: Why not turn to a skills training model? *American Journal of Occupational Therapy, 49,* 721–723.

Peloquin, S. M. (1995b). The fullness of empathy: Reflections and illustrations. *American Journal of Occupational Therapy, 49,* 24–31.

Peloquin, S. M. (1996a). Art: An occupation with promise for developing empathy. *American Journal of Occupational Therapy, 50,* 655–661.

Peloquin, S. M. (1996b). The Issue Is—Now that we have managed care, shall we inspire it? *American Journal of Occupational Therapy, 50,* 455–459.

Peloquin, S. M. (1996c). Brief or New—Using the arts to enhance confluent learning. *American Journal of Occupational Therapy, 50,* 148–151.

Peloquin, S. M. (1998). The therapeutic relationship. In M. E. Neistadt & E. B. Crepeau (Eds.), *Willard and Spackman's occupational therapy* (9th ed., pp. 105–119). Philadelphia: Lippincott.

Peloquin, S. M., & Davidson, D. A. (1993). Brief or New—Interpersonal skills for practice: An elective course. *American Journal of Occupational Therapy, 47,* 260–264.

Peloquin, S. M., & Shelton, M. (1997). Doubletakes. *Revista OT, 62,* 6.

Suggested Readings

Adamson, B. J., Hunt, A. E., Harris, L. M., & Hummel, J. (1998). Occupational therapists' perceptions of their undergraduate preparation for the workplace. *British Journal of Occupational Therapy, 61,* 173–179.

American Occupational Therapy Association. (1997). Philosophy of education. *American Journal of Occupational Therapy, 51,* 867.

Bolles, R. N. (1981). *The three boxes of life.* Berkeley, CA: Ten Speed Press.

Gardner, J. (1963). *Self-renewal.* New York: Harper & Row.

Ilott, I., & Kenyon, J. (1997). Bridging the gap: Employment and education: Part I: An evaluation of an in-service course. *British Journal of Occupational Therapy, 60,* 301–304.

Interaction between education and practice. (1996). *OT Practice, 1*(8), 9–10.

Kenyon, J., & Ilott, I. (1997). Bridging the gap: Employment and education: Part II: Education into practice. *British Journal of Occupational Therapy, 60,* 343–346.

King, L. J. (1986). Competence and credibility: A challenge to professional self-discipline. *Occupational Therapy Forum, 1*(6), 13–14.

Lunt, A. (1996). Is fieldwork training or education? *British Journal of Occupational Therapy, 59*, 586.

Lyons, M. (1996). Process over person? Occupational therapy students' fieldwork experience of people in psychiatric settings. *Disability and Rehabilitation, 18*(4), 197–204.

Martin M., & Edwards, L. (1998). Peer learning on fieldwork placements. *British Journal of Occupational Therapy, 61*, 249–252.

McClellan, M., & Cantu, C. (1997). Developing a collaborative teaching model. *OT Practice, 2*(11), 47–49.

McNurlen, G. (1997). Education: A growing practice area. *OT Practice, 2*(6), 40–43.

Peters, T. J., & Waterman, R. H. (1984). *In search of excellence*. New York: Warner.

Ravetz, C., & Granell, C. (1996). The establishment of occupational therapy clinics within and educational setting: A report. *British Journal of Occupational Therapy, 59*, 503–505.

Renwick, R., Cockburn, L., Colantonio, A., & Friedland, J. (1996). Preparing students for practice in a changing community environment: An innovative course. *Occupational Therapy International, 3*(4), 262–273.

Stancliff, B. L. (1996). Giving structure to new responsibilities, tasks. *OT Practice, 1*(10), 15–19.

INVITED ARTICLES

Establishing Links With Clinical and Management Functions

Beatriz C. Abreu

Beatriz C. Abreu, PhD, OTR, FAOTA, is Director of Occupational Therapy, Transitional Learning Center at Galveston, and Clinical Professor, University of Texas Medical Branch at Galveston, Galveston, Texas.

Scholarly activity and research transcend the boundaries inherent in the discrete roles and functions of practitioners. In this article, the author provides a brief discussion aimed to expand the utility of scholarly activity by linking management and research. The author discusses the links between competence and systematic inquiry and between simplification and transformation strategies. The author also makes conclusions about clinical and educational implications.

In many respects, the occupations, roles, and functions we perform in our workplace define us. They give us an identity, focus our educational agendas, and foster participation in academically based education. Postprofessional education focuses on research and advanced clinical skills to enhance and enrich the profession of occupational therapy and the discipline of occupational science. Practitioners who seek career advancement and enrichment return to academically based postprofessional education for specialized training to develop research and scholarly competence (Abreu & Blount, 1993). Many postprofessional programs present research and scholarly activity as discrete functions with limited relevance, which results in a practice that is elitist. This is unfortunate because this elitism creates a perception of research that is mystifying, irrelevant, and inaccessible. Occupational therapy supports actions to create partnerships to combine resources for beneficial and meaningful connections such as linking research and management (Peloquin & Abreu, 1996). Linking managerial and research functions can change the perception of how to teach research.

A manager is any person whose role is systematically to ensure, monitor, and regulate work, organizations, production, and operations (American Occupational Therapy Association, 1993; Schell & Slater, 1998). A researcher is any person whose role is systematically to investigate phenomena by using methods such as observation, reasoning, analysis, and interpretation (Gutman & Mortera, 1997; Mosey, 1989). Although the roles of both the manager and the researcher are discrete functions, we need to acknowledge that their roles are complex and multidimensional and frequently overlap. Both the manager and the researcher, however, use data as information in their decision-making processes.

Linking Management and Research Through Competence and Systematic Inquiry

Management and research functions are linked through the process of competence and systematic inquiry. In today's health care environment, both the manager and researcher must increase competence that will improve job behaviors and productivity. *Competence* is a complex and evolving set of cognitive, affective, and psychomotor abilities that determines how a person performs his or her job duties (Youngstrom, 1998). One can view competence as a nonhierarchical weave of three strands (Figure 1). The strands are knowledge, skills, and attitudes (Abreu, Peloquin, & Ottenbacher, 1998). Both the manager and the researcher use the same strands in their weave of competence. The knowledge and the attitude strands are somewhat similar. Even the skills strand, which is different, has some common traits. Therefore, the link between management and research competencies is strong. The capabilities of individual managers and researchers from novice to expert may affect the link.

A second link involves the scholarly process of systematic inquiry. Mosey (1998) defined this process as a series of intellectual activities directed toward synthesizing, categorizing, defining, and collecting information or data to create sound and practical information. Both managers and researchers engage in this form of investigation because they must process data in an accurate, critical, and thorough manner. However, the researcher undertakes basic or applied scientific investigations to formulate or refine theories or to find a solution to an immediate practical problem (Mosey, 1996). The manager, on the other hand, undertakes practical investigations such as program evaluations, quality improvement, and outcome research. The researcher uses scientific inquiry to discover, expand, generate, and test applications of knowledge. Scientific inquiry is the broad undertaking within which research serves as a tool (Mosey, 1996). Managers are collaborators and critical research consumers. They can help the staff members to integrate research into the clinical reasoning process (Tickle-Degnen, 1999). Both managers and researchers use research findings as a basis for improving clinical practice (Rosenberg & Donald, 1995).

Linking Management and Research Through Simplification and Transformation Strategies

Effective management requires strategies to accomplish outcomes and goals. These strategies are organized rules that guide behavior. Simplification of clinical documentation and transformation of clinical goals are two strategies that have helped to interface management and research in clinical practice. Clinical documentation includes daily notes, progress reports, evaluations, and discharge reports. Simplification of this process makes documentation easier and less complicated at the operational and technical level and can be accomplished by creating electronic records with built-in documentation templates that provide a means to improve the quality and the utility of the information about the services provided. Not only are electronic records are used to develop efficient departmental operations, but they also can make integrating management and research easier. Information from these managerial records may help to establish

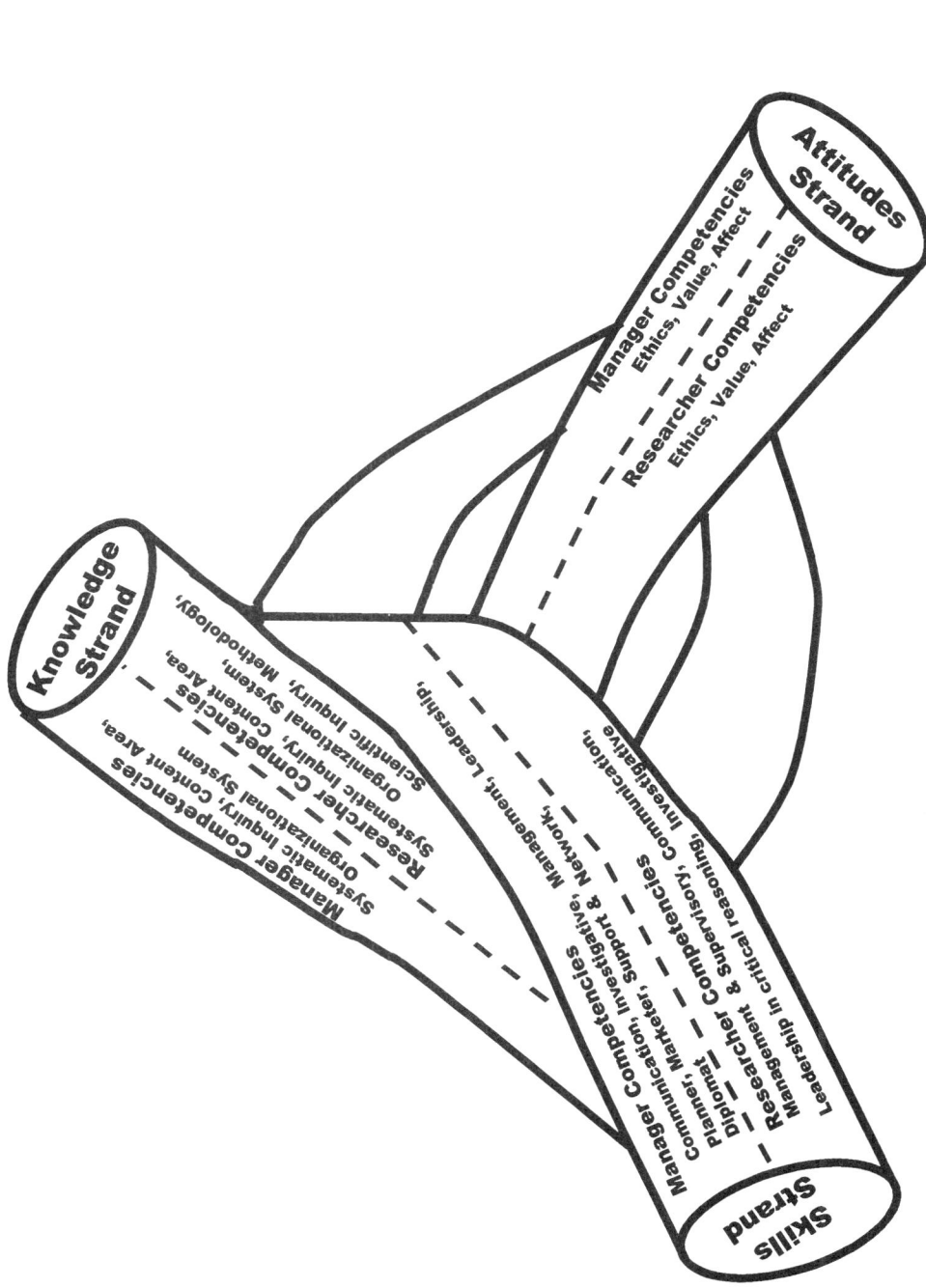

Figure 1. Weave of researcher-associated and manager-associated competencies. Note. From "Competence in Scientific Inquiry and Research," by B. C. Abreu, S. M. Peloquin, and K. Ottenbacher, 1998, American Journal of Occupational Therapy, 52, p. 756. Copyright 1998 by The American Occupational Therapy Association, Inc.

a research database. However, we must remember to observe all ethical and legal guidelines by protecting the client's confidentiality and obtaining consent. Electronic records can improve the documentation of a client's direct health care services (Dwyer, 1999).

In the clinic, occupational therapy managers must understand the culture of the institution in which they work. Occupational therapy managers must create opportunities for themselves and others to meet their personal goals, the client's goals, and the organization's goals. Transformation of clinical goals is the action of understanding and changing the nature or structure of operations to facilitate the organizational, departmental, or personal missions. Three transformation strategies can link management and research. The first strategy is to establish and implement a department mission statement, the second is to decentralize the management of the department, and the third is to integrate information into an organized system that integrates quantitative and qualitative client data to preserve the individual perspective of the client receiving occupational therapy services.

The first transformation strategy the manager often uses is that of establishing and implementing organizational, departmental, and personal goals that include scholarly and research endeavors. For example, our institution's goals are threefold:

1. To provide quality direct care service
2. To provide quality clinical education
3. To conduct systematic investigations to support clinical outcomes and evidenced-based practice

To accomplish these goals, the manager incorporates these missions into the individual job descriptions and provides a time frame in which to fulfill them. Making research part of the job has demystified it through systematic investigation of the evaluations, interventions, and daily reports.

The second transformation strategy is to establish a nonhierarchical management structure by decentralizing the department through a redistribution of leadership according to staff member knowledge, skills, and values. This strategy requires awareness of the emotional and cognitive issues that managers and subordinates face (Abreu, 1997). Decentralization empowers expert and novice staff members by rotating responsibilities. In a nonhierarchical department, all members improve their performance while pursuing the prescribed goals of excellent direct care, clinical education, and research. Staff member discussion of required readings (journal clubs) has been quite successful. Professional consultations and mentoring by academicians has likewise been effective.

The third transformation strategy is to interface qualitative and quantitative client data to preserve the individuality and humanistic perspective of the client receiving occupational therapy services (Abreu, 1998a, 1998b). Encouraging versatility of data collection systems has helped us to capture the individual dimension of both clients and staff members. Various computer programs are available to assist staff members in the reduction, display, and analysis of information. The guidelines for appraising the usefulness and suitability of the clinical data involve answering questions and explaining phenomena related to the clients, staff members, and the institution served.

Reflections on the roles of the manager and researcher can demystify the research process. All practitioners must use data appropriately in their attempt to optimize intervention and, therefore, must develop research competencies in all occupational therapy roles. The implication is that research is a clinical requirement and an ethical obligation. Managers can foster the research process by using simplification and transformation strategies. Research is not a substitute for clinical reasoning (Tickle-Degnen, 1999). Clinical reasoning transcends research and evidence-based practice. Educators can contribute to the linking of management and research by creating a climate that acknowledges research as a nonlinear process and by developing a curriculum that focuses on research skills across all occupational therapy roles. ▪

References

Abreu, B. C. (1997). Interdisciplinary leadership. *Occupational Therapy Practice, 2,* 20–25.

Abreu, B. C. (1998a). Additional uses for data. In J. Hinojosa & P. Kramer (Eds.), *Occupational therapy evaluation: Obtaining and interpreting data* (pp. 213–234). Bethesda, MD: American Occupational Therapy Association.

Abreu, B. C. (1998b). The quadraphonic approach: Holistic rehabilitation for brain injury. In N. Katz (Ed.), *Cognition and occupation in rehabilitation: Cognitive models for intervention in occupational therapy* (pp. 51–97). Bethesda, MD: American Occupational Therapy Association.

Abreu, B. C., & Blount, M.-L. F. (1993). The Issue Is—Academically based education versus continuing education: The best way to go. *American Journal of Occupational Therapy, 47,* 82–88.

Abreu, B. C., Peloquin, S. M., & Ottenbacher, K. (1998). Competence in scientific inquiry and research. *American Journal of Occupational Therapy, 52,* 751–758.

American Occupational Therapy Association. (1993). Occupational therapy roles. *American Journal of Occupational Therapy, 47,* 1087–1099.

Dwyer, C. (1999). Ideas and trends: Medical informatics and health care computing. *Annals of Internal Medicine, 130,* 170–172.

Gutman, S. A., & Mortera, M. (1997). The Issue Is—Applied scientific inquiry: An answer to managed care's challenge? *American Journal of Occupational Therapy, 51,* 704–709.

Mosey, A. C. (1989). Editorial—The proper focus of scientific inquiry in occupational therapy: Frames of reference. *Occupational Therapy Journal of Research, 9,* 195–201.

Mosey, A. C. (1996). *Applied scientific inquiry in the health professions: An epistemological orientation* (2nd ed.). Bethesda, MD: American Occupational Therapy Association.

Mosey, A. C. (1998). The competent scholar. *American Journal of Occupational Therapy, 52,* 760–764.

Peloquin, S., & Abreu, B. C. (1996). The Issue Is—The academic and clinical worlds: Shall we make meaningful connections. *American Journal of Occupational Therapy, 50,* 588–591.

Rosenberg, W., & Donald, A. (1995). Evidence-based medicine: An approach to clinical problem solving. *British Medical Journal, 310,* 1122–1126.

Schell, B. A. B., & Slater, D. Y. (1998). Management competencies required of administrative and clinical practitioners in the new millennium. *American Journal of Occupational Therapy, 52,* 744–750.

Tickle-Degnen, L. (1999). Evidence-Based Practice Forum—Organizing, evaluating, and using evidence in occupational therapy practice. *American Journal of Occupational Therapy, 53,* 537–539.

Youngstrom, M. J. (1998). Evolving competence in the practitioner role. *American Journal of Occupational Therapy, 52,* 716–720.

INVITED ARTICLES

Establishing Links With Graduate Education

Janette Schkade

Janette Schkade, PhD, OTR, FAOTA, is Professor and Dean, Texas Woman's University, School of Occupational Therapy, Denton, Texas.

Development of the profession of occupational therapy in part depends on scholarly discourse. This article proposes that graduate education is the most likely place that skills necessary for engagement in scholarly discourse will develop. Skill in presenting ideas in a public forum for critical examination is one mechanism for fostering the ability to engage in scholarly discourse. This article presents examples of strategies that Texas Woman's University uses in graduate education to promote scholarly engagement and offers suggestions for faculty members, scholarly critics, and students.

According to Yerxa (1982), occupational therapy has historically ignored scholarly discourse. Some notable exceptions include the discussion regarding pluralism versus monism of Mosey (1985) and Christiansen (1990). Another exception was the dialogue between Mosey (1992, 1993) and the faculty members from the University of Southern California (Clark et al., 1993) regarding the partition between occupational science and occupational therapy. More recently, a series of articles debated the merits of Fidler's (1996) model of lifestyle performance and the subsequent dialogue that followed (Hengel, 1997; Hocking & Whiteford, 1997, 1998; Velde, Gerney, Trompetter, & Amory, 1997).

Dunn, Schulz, Schulz, Honaker, and Wiley (1999) traced the history of their own ability to discuss scholarly issues through their experiences as students in a doctoral program. Scholarly discourse requires a public presentation of ideas, either in an oral presentation or in print. Public disclosure of ideas then allows comment and critique, which leads to modification, refinement, and thoughtful discussion. In my experience, the motivation and ability to engage in scholarly inquiry and exchange is a learned skill.

The comments that follow have three premises:
1. Maturity as a profession will depend, in part, on the development of a body of knowledge through research and scholarly activities.
2. Scholarly discourse is essential to the expansion, elaboration, and therapeutic utility of that body of knowledge.
3. Skill to engage in scholarly discourse is most likely to be promoted at the level of graduate or postbaccalaureate education.

The educator faces some challenges when engaging students in the process of scholarly discourse. The educator must overcome these challenges if students are to participate in this discourse successfully. One challenge is that students often believe that only others can engage in scholarly discourse. We must confront the myth that only those in the highest echelons of scholarly pursuits can be a part of the scholarly effort, and we must empower students with the belief that they, too, are capable. Anxiety about participation in public arenas is a related concern for the novice scholar. The educator must carefully facilitate and mentor the student's ability to risk public consideration of his or her scholarly ideas and products.

Strategies for Engaging Students in Scholarly Discourse

At Texas Woman's University, we have used three strategies to promote student engagement in public scholarly discourse:

1. Students present their scholarly work in a public forum.
2. Respected scholars in the profession offer public critique and discussion.
3. Students role-play the critic function.

The first two strategies have been exemplified in events featuring professional master's degree students (master of occupational therapy [MOT]) and doctoral students. Students in our Pi Theta Epsilon chapter in Dallas, Texas, established the "Celebration of Scholarship" in 1993, a tradition that continues today. The presenters have been primarily professional master's degree students. Our MOT students must produce a scholarly work as part of the requirements for all master's degrees. The celebration is a 1-day event with platform and poster presentations. Students select an invited scholar who presents a keynote address and then comments on student presentations. The goal of this event is that students will come away from the experience with a positive view of presenting their work in a forum in which they subject it to public scrutiny. The invited scholars are selected with care. They must be persons who are known as scholars in the profession and who have an interest in promoting scholarship in beginning scholars. To date, the scholars have included Suzanne Peloquin, Jerry Johnson, Jennifer Angelo, Nedra Gillette, Jim Hinojosa, Wendy Wood, and Kathlyn Reed.

A second major event was our first Occupational Adaptation Symposium in March 1998. The symposium featured the scholarly work of our doctoral students. Entitled "Weaving Ordinary Acts into Extraordinary Outcomes," this 1 1/2 days of student presentations consisted of much more advanced and conceptual work than that which the MOT students presented. We divided the papers into three categories:

1. Enriching the theoretical foundations of occupation and adaptation
2. Person–environment interactive process in various contexts
3. Occupational adaptation as a therapeutic tool

Doctoral faculty members presented concept papers to set the stage for each of the groupings. A keynote speaker outside of occupational therapy, geographer Graham Rowles, was one of the discussants. Three occupational therapy scholars who had been consultants in the developmental stages of the doctoral program (Anne Henderson, Lela Llorens, and Kathlyn Reed) returned to discuss the scholarship.

A third strategy we use with postprofessional master's degree and doctoral students has been to place the student in the role of critic. Research proposals written for a culminating assignment in research courses provide the context. Students are "committee chairs" or "committee members." The students then have the responsibility of reading and critiquing the proposals and conducting a simulated proposal defense. This experience helps the students to understand the function of the faculty member directing and critiquing a student's scholarly work and to develop an appreciation for the importance of the defense process and the rigor required.

Suggestions for Faculty Members, Critics, and Students

Development of the capacity for scholarly discourse in graduate students suggests considerations for all parties involved: faculty members, scholarly critics, and students. Faculty members must remember that they are dealing with a developmental process. We cannot overestimate the importance of an appropriate level of challenge. The faculty member must be satisfied with a presentation that is less than exquisitely polished and recognize the performance rudiments that reflect an emerging skill. Focusing on the intellectual development of the student and not on the presentation itself is helpful.

Critiquing scholars must remember the developmental process. When a scholar provides a level of criticism that the student can manage at a particular developmental level, then that is a gift to the student. Scholars must communicate their comments in an understandable fashion that enhances the student's understanding rather than dazzling the student with the scholar's own intellectual prowess.

Students must grapple with the elements that produce anxiety. They must prepare well and plan for contingencies, such as technical difficulties, unexpected reductions in time allotted, and so forth. Students should recognize and accept the fact that "things can go wrong." The unexpected question or comment from the critic that elicits a momentary cognitive blank is a common occurrence. The identification, at a much later time, of an appropriate comment or insight is an experience that can plague even advanced scholars. Students who remember that they are in the process of developing scholarly skills for a lifetime are more likely to view the event and its associated personal costs as worthwhile.

A cadre of thoughtful scholars willing to share their work with members of the profession is essential to our grounding as an evidence-based intervention. Development of that group of scholars requires that faculty members and scholar critics identify persons with the basic intellect and talent necessary.

Guiding the exposure of those persons to culminate in the emergence of skills associated with scholarly discourse constitutes an important role for graduate educators. ∎

References

Christiansen, C. H. (1990). The perils of plurality. *Occupational Therapy Journal of Research, 10,* 259–265.

Clark, F., Zemke, R., Frank, G., Parham, D., Neville-Jan, A., Hendricks, C., Carson, M., Fazio, L. & Abreu, B. (1993). The Issue Is—Dangers inherent in the partition of occupational therapy and occupational science. *American Journal of Occupational Therapy, 47,* 184–186.

Dunn, E., Schulz, E. K., Schulz, C. H., Honaker, D. & Wiley, A. M. (1999). The Issue Is—The importance of scholarly debate in occupational therapy. *American Journal of Occupational Therapy, 53,* 398–400.

Fidler, G. S. (1996). Life-style performance: From profile to conceptual model. *American Journal of Occupational Therapy, 50,* 139–147.

Hengel, J. (1997). Letters to the Editor—Criticism of Fidler's model debated. *American Journal of Occupational Therapy, 51,* 710.

Hocking, C., & Whiteford, G. (1997). The Issue Is—What are the criteria for development of occupational therapy theory? A response to Fidler's life style performance model. *American Journal of Occupational Therapy, 51,* 154–157.

Hocking, C., & Whiteford, G. (1998). Letters to the Editor—Authors' response [to Hengel, 1998]. *American Journal of Occupational Therapy, 51,* 710.

Mosey, A. C. (1985). A monistic or pluralistic approach to professional identity? 1985 Eleanor Clarke Slagle lecture. *American Journal of Occupational Therapy, 39,* 504–509.

Mosey, A. C. (1992). The Issue Is—Partition of occupational science and occupational therapy. *American Journal of Occupational Therapy, 46,* 851–853.

Mosey, A. C. (1993). The Issue Is—Partition of occupational science and occupational therapy: Sorting out some issues. *American Journal of Occupational Therapy, 47,* 751–754.

Velde, B. P., Gerney, A., Trompetter, L., & Amory, M. A. (1997). The Issue Is—Fidler's life style performance model: Why we disagree with Hocking and Whiteford's critique. *American Journal of Occupational Therapy, 51,* 784–787.

Yerxa, E. J. (1982). The Issue—A response to testing and measurement in occupational therapy: A review of current practice with special emphasis on the Southern California Sensory Integration Tests. *American Journal of Occupational Therapy, 36,* 399–404.

Information for Authors

The *Innovations in Occupational Therapy Education* (IOTE) Editor invites manuscript submissions that conform to its aim and scope without regard to the professional affiliations of authors. Five types of contributions are considered:

1. Full-length or feature articles
2. Brief reports
3. Letters to the editor
4. Book, monograph, and technology reviews
5. Commentaries

Guidelines for preparing and submitting manuscripts are outlined subsequently. Manuscripts that do not substantially comply with these guidelines will be returned to the author(s) without consideration.

Manuscript Preparation

All manuscripts should be prepared according to the IOTE Requirements for Submission of Manuscripts and Disks.

General Style and Format Considerations

Authors should prepare manuscripts in accordance with the latest (1994) edition of the *Publication Manual of the American Psychological Association* (APA). Neither the American Occupational Therapy Association nor IOTE editorial staff members can assume responsibility for statements or opinions expressed by authors. Authors are strongly encouraged to consult the APA publication manual (4th edition), for more detailed advice on the preparation of manuscripts.

Specific Guidelines by Type of Contribution

Feature Articles

Full-length research articles should generally not exceed 4,000 words (15 double-spaced typewritten pages, including tables, references, and figures). Each article must be accompanied by an abstract that clearly, completely, and succinctly summarizes the material that follows. Abstracts of empirical studies should be 100 to 150 words in length; theoretical articles should be 75 to 100 words. Each article must be accompanied by a one-sentence explanation of how this work will benefit occupational therapy practitioners or the practice of occupational therapy. Pages should be numbered consecutively (except for figures) in the following order: title page (page 1), abstract (page 2), text (beginning on page 3), references (new page after text), appendices (each on a new page), and tables and figures (each on separate pages). This arrangement is necessary for copy processing and does not represent how the manuscript will appear in print. Identify each manuscript page (except the figures) by typing the first 2 to 3 words from the title in the upper right-hand corner above the page number.

The title page should contain the authors' names, affiliations, complete mailing address, e-mail address, and telephone and fax numbers. It should include the one-sentence explanation of the work's relevance to occupational therapy. The title page should list acknowledgments, grant or contract support, and information concerning previous presentation of the material at symposia or conferences.

Briefs

IOTE will publish expanded descriptions of innovative approaches to fieldwork instructional methods and research in education outcomes. Submitted manuscripts in this category must be limited to 1,000 words and be as succinct, accurate, and informative as possible.

Reviews

Book, monograph, journal, and technology reviews are limited to 500 words and should include an objective and substantive appraisal of the item's merit. Provide the names of authors, the title in full, the publisher and city, the date or frequency of publication, the number of pages, and the purchase or subscription price.

Letters to the Editor

Letters must be limited to 500 words and should provide thoughtful scientific criticism, rebuttal, or personal data relating to research articles or commentary published in IOTE. No more than five citations and references can be included. Unless specifically indicated to the contrary, all letters will be assumed to be for publication and will be subject to the same editorial revision policies as other manuscripts.

Commentaries

Scholarly discussion of emerging educational issues will be considered. Submitted manuscripts in this category typically are limited to 2,000 words and must be as succinct, accurate, and informative as possible. In some cases, the Editor may publish a counterpoint or opposing view commentary to stimulate thought and discussion.

Manuscript Submission

Submit manuscripts in *quadruplicate* to the Editor, whose address follows. A cover letter should accompany articles, abstracts, or review manuscripts indicating that the material is not currently under consideration for publication elsewhere. The letter should designate the name of the corresponding author, if different from the senior (first) author.

Authors should retain copies of all material submitted to guard against loss. IOTE cannot assume responsibility for lost manuscripts. If copyrighted material is included in the manuscript, evidence of written permission to reproduce said material must be enclosed with the cover letter. Manuscripts will be acknowledged on receipt. After preliminary review, they will be sent to members of the editorial board. Notification of disposition may take between 2 and 3 months after acknowledgment. Accepted manuscripts will be published only on receipt of signed copyright assignment forms from the authors along with a hard copy and a copy of the entire manuscript on a floppy disk. The copyright so conveyed includes any and all subsidiary forms of publication, including electronic media.

Authors will have the opportunity to review typeset page proofs of the manuscript before publication. Page proofs MUST be returned within 48 hours of receipt—they are for correction only and not for rewrite. Delayed return of page proofs will result in forfeiture of the author's opportunity for prepublication review. IOTE reserves the right to make or request editorial changes in all manuscripts accepted for publication.

Address all editorial correspondence and manuscripts to the Editor, Patricia A. Crist, PhD, OTR/L, FAOTA, IOTE, Department of Occupational Therapy, Rangos School of Health Sciences, Duquesne University, 600 Forbes Avenue, Pittsburgh, Pennsylvania 15282-0020; Internet address (for inquiries or questions only): crist@duq2.cc.duq.edu.

Checklist

(Consult the following instructions before you submit your manuscript package to the American Occupational Therapy Association [AOTA])

1. Print manuscript on one side of standard-sized (8.5 × 11 in. [22 × 28 cm]) white paper.
2. Use either Times Roman or Courier 12-point typeface.
3. Double-space between all lines of the manuscript, including title, headings, footnotes, quotations, references, figure captions, and all parts of tables.
4. Use one space between words. Eliminate all instances of 2 spaces.
5. Leave margins of at least 1 in. (2.54 cm) at the left, right, top, and bottom of every page.
6. Use the flush-left style or ragged right margin of line justification.
7. Indicate a new paragraph by using 2 hard returns, rather than by using tabs or spaces.
8. Turn off the hyphenation function so that no words are divided at the end of the line.
9. Number pages consecutively, beginning with the title page, in the upper right-hand corner.
10. Spell out abbreviations and acronyms the first time they appear in text, follow with abbreviation in parentheses, and use the abbreviation consistently throughout the remainder of the text. Eliminate unnecessary abbreviations.
11. Use generic drug and equipment names; insert proprietary names in parentheses at the point of first mention; if it is necessary to use a trademark, include the manufacturer's name, city, and state.
12. Express weights and measures in standard and metric units; express temperatures in degrees Fahrenheit and in degrees centigrade.
13. Include page numbers in text for all quotations.
14. Cite references in both the text and in the reference list; make sure the entries agree in spelling and in date.
15. Spell out journal titles completely.
16. Alphabetize references in the reference list by the author's surname.
17. Provide inclusive page numbers for all articles or chapters in books.
18. Provide written permission for all materials obtained from other publishers. Include the page numbers of your manuscript to which the permission refers. Provide model releases for any full-face or partial-face photos of persons. Sample release forms are available from AOTA.
19. Provide clearly labeled camera-ready art for all illustrations, including photographs, and mark the locations for placement within the manuscript.

20. Retain a copy of your manuscript, paper files, art, and electronic files. Do not send your only copies.
21. Please understand that your submission is final copy. Pages reviewed later for proofing are for correction only and not for rewrite.

Art Requirements

If possible, submit art on disk and indicate software version used to create information.

Line Drawings, Tables, and Graphs

1. Provide crisp, clean originals in black on smooth white paper.
2. Remove unnecessary smudges.
3. Do not send poor-quality "patchy" photocopies. Be sure photocopies include the complete page and that the page is evenly reproduced.
4. Do not enclose faxes of artwork because these do not reproduce well.

Photographs

1. Send either color or black-and-white photographs.
2. Use either color or black-and-white prints in the largest format possible (4 × 6 in. or 8 × 10 in.).
3. Use color or black-and-white 35-mm slides or transparencies.

Submit a self-addressed, stamped postcard with your manuscript. On the blank side, provide the authors and title of the manuscript you are submitting for review.

Effective and economical use of your word-processing file depends on its being consistently prepared. Please follow the APA guidelines for preparing a manuscript (chapter 4). You are responsible for ensuring that the electronic files on your submitted diskettes exactly match the hardcopy printout of the submitted manuscript.

Final Manuscript Submission Only (accepted for publication)

(If your article is accepted for publication you will have to meet the following additional requirement when submitting your final edited draft to the Editor)

1. Provide clearly labeled diskettes with your name, telephone number, and file names in WordPerfect 5.1 or Microsoft Word on a 3.5-inch high density diskette (1.44–2 MB).
2. Label your envelope with "disk enclosed" to ensure proper handling by post office personnel.
3. Be sure that all earlier versions of your manuscript are deleted from the disk.